What better gift?

The collected wisdoms

proven and enthusiastically shared

by individuals who have learned

to make life wonderful!

the SHORT COURSE TO

Mental Wealth

THROUGH A NEWER WAY OF THINKING

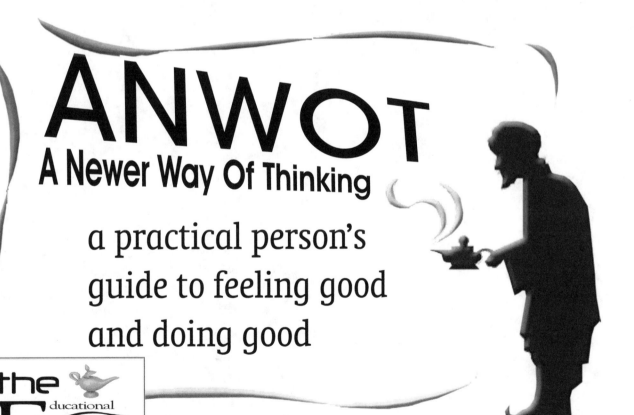

ANWOT

A Newer Way Of Thinking

a practical person's
guide to feeling good
and doing good

the
Educational
Community
inc.

DONALD PET, M.D.

THE SHORT COURSE TO MENTAL WEALTH

through

A Newer Way of Thinking = ANWOT

DONALD PET, M.D.

A practical person's guide to feeling good and doing good

Make this your most important read ever!

1. Become your own best friend, lifelong.
2. Strengthen *self*-mastery: free your mind from the prejudices of its early masters as you become your own genie.
3. Attain peace of mind; become a force for world peace.

Peace of Mind and **Peace in the World** are universal common prayers. A Newer Way of Thinking is a self-study guide containing the mental skills that others have shown "work." The ANWOT skills will empower you to answer such prayers. You have been taught the three R's and how to make a living; you are now ready for a graduate course in making your life wonderful.

The Short Course to Mental Wealth consists of eight easy-to-learn sections containing approximately ten pages each. This educational program along with the full course, A Newer Way of Thinking, is FREE on the Internet: **www.anwot.org**.

The Educational Community is a 501(c)(3) nonprofit corporation whose mission is to promote the newer ways of thinking we require if we choose to survive and thrive in the new nuclear age.

THE SHORT COURSE TO MENTAL WEALTH
A PRACTICAL PERSONS GUIDE TO FEELING GOOD AND DOING GOOD

BY DONALD PET, M.D.

ALSO AUTHOR OF:

A NEWER WAY OF THINKING
HOW TO SURVIVE AND THRIVE IN THE NUCLEAR AGE

For information, contact:

Donald Pet, M.D.
c/o The Educational Community, Inc.
235 East River Drive, #1107
East Hartford, CT 06108
Visit: anwot.org

ISBN: 978-0-615-22576-0   Softcover Edition
ISBN: 978-0-981-93310-8   Hardcover Edition

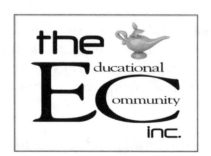

Printed in the United States of America
The Educational Community, Inc. with BookMasters, Inc.

In consultation with:
American Photos, Graphics & Designs Publishing, LLC
www.PicturesToArt.com

The Short Course To Mental Wealth

About the Author

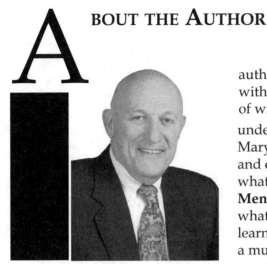

Donald Pet, M.D.: I see myself more as editor than author, for it has been my good fortune to walk and talk with inspirational mentors and bathe in so many fountains of wisdom as part of my life's education – including undergraduate and psychiatric training at Johns Hopkins, Maryland Medical School, my professional career, friends, and especially former patients who shared their insights to what works. I claim the originality of **The Short Course to Mental Wealth** and **A Newer Way of Thinking** is joining what others have generously provided into an easily learned expandable self-education curriculum; I credit a multitude of unnamed heroes[1] with the creation of the powerful wisdoms ANWOT offers.

I'm especially proud of my efforts in having created the first Educational Community in a prison setting at the Lexington, Kentucky Federal Narcotics Hospital/Prison, in the Connecticut Department of Mental Health substance abuse program, and in a private practice treatment program. I learned that, given the opportunity to teach our *self* and with motivation, people can attain their most fulfilling goals. If heroin addicted "life-style criminals" can re-invent themselves and become effective counselors to others, if chronically depressed or otherwise mentally impaired persons can re-establish their lives as enthusiastic productive citizens, why not the rest of us?

I have acquired expertise in community health through my professional career. I authored over 5 million dollars in federal grants to create and direct a multi-modality substance abuse treatment program serving the greater Hartford, CT area and thereafter the CT Alcohol and Drug Training Center. It provided education and staff development to law enforcement, judicial, and treatment personnel among others; I have given hundreds of public presentations. Achievements include chairing a committee authorized by the legislature to interview experts on marihuana and submit a report. With the cooperation of the Commissioner of Mental Health, the legislature authorized the hiring of counselors based on life experience as an alternative to the standard academic credentials; this allowed recovered addicts to obtain State jobs.

Now celebrating over 50 years of marriage, joys from my three sons and daughters-in-laws, seven grandchildren, and having attained financial well-being through successful investments, my current enthusiasm is to sow what I have reaped. I do believe we have, in our lifetime, entered a Nuclear Era in which our troubles will reach unimaginable harm unless we spread *the newer way of thinking* that is within our grasp. Retirement has provided me the opportunity to direct my energy to what I believe is now the greatest and most neglected threat to humanity; the management of destructive aggression. *Each one, teach one.* What better way to give back than to become *one* offering to teach *one*? Please join me; become *one* too.

I have created a 501 (c)(3) non-profit corporation, The Educational Community, Inc., to develop and popularize education in the newer way of thinking Albert Einstein told us we require if we are to prevent humankind from using its best to do its worst. I am especially appreciative if you join me in growing ANWOT for our mutual benefit, for those we love, and those whom we may never meet.

---

[1] I choose to identify one favorite inspirational teacher and role model, Jerome D. Frank, M.D., Ph.D., professor of psychiatry at Johns Hopkins (deceased); author of <u>Persuasion and Healing</u>, and <u>Sanity & Survival</u>, <u>Psychological Aspects of War and Peace</u>.

INTRODUCTION █

Mental wealth is the means by which we make our wishes become a reality. We attain mental wealth by accumulating the wisdoms that empower us to become our own genie. Genies make wishes come true in return for being freed from their prison. I became my own genie through the mental wealth I acquired from my many teachers. They freed themselves from the prejudices of fate and circumstance to become masters of their own minds. They successfully created a fulfilled life. Through their wisdom, I have created a wonderful life; so can you.

As my mental wealth was gladly provided to me by many others, I can now fulfill my duty to share my riches. I enthusiastically do so through two books, this *Short Course* and the full course, *A Newer Way of Thinking*. **Mental wealth, unlike physical wealth, is not limited in quantity and our personal genie is not limited to the traditional three wishes.** My wealth grows by each degree you become your own genie and join me in making our most universal wishes a reality: peace of mind and world peace. Please accept my gift for our mutual benefit.

Mental wealth is comprised of individual strands of wisdom or "strens" which we make stronger, like our strands of muscle, through exercise. A *stren or unit of mental wealth* is any idea, insight, wisdom, and/or experience that contributes to our well-being. The word was created by a group of mental health professionals following a lecture by anthropologist Margaret Mead. She pointed out that our language biases our thinking towards negative interpretations. Our manner of thinking, like a computer lacking an adequate word processing program, remains limited until we upgrade our mind for maturity. Working together, our collection of strens totals more than the sum of their individual value. As a dedicated stren seeker throughout my nearly complete life, I have amassed an extensive collection which is yours for the taking. Make the word "stren" an important addition to your vocabulary.

Acquiring wealth beyond our dreams is possible for every ordinary person who is willing to study and put into practice what others have shown "works." The first step to mental wealth is creating a spark through the simple belief that "**I can.**" Thereafter add **work, patience, direction**, and the **risk-taking** needed to challenge the habitual way of thinking that no longer works. These five ingredients are either already in our possession or are abundantly available and easy to obtain, as will be explained. Realize that we don't need money or physical wealth, special genes, unusual intelligence, good looks, titles or connections, and not even good health. Luck is always helpful and absolutely zero magic is required. My proof of this is my direct and indirect observation of many persons who lack the above "silver spoons" yet enthusiastically and convincingly lead a glorious life. And I have seen many individuals who have many or all of the usually ascribed material "wants" who don't make it; they are well represented among those who commit suicide. Indeed, the wealthiest person I've met was by my observation (and his), among the most miserable.

You'll get the idea and inspiration each time you read "the strength stren," (literally *the mental strength skill*) provided on page 7. Let's focus on the strens shown to be effective by joyous fulfilled individuals, many burdened with the severest of hardships and without the "goodies" others traditionally seek.

The strens I claim and here share are the powerful mental skills that others have shown create the results they desire. Strens are available in abundance in our commonly shared media and literature. I offer my collection to you in a *free* Internet book, *A Newer Way of Thinking*, at **www.anwot.org**. I owe this collection to my privileged education, including training in psychiatry at Johns Hopkins; the opportunity to learn from others, especially patients who have willingly, even enthusiastically offered their insights to well-being; and my continuing zeal as a life-time "collector." Some will find the book's 397 pages a bit tedious, so I have written this practical "quick fix," *also free*, for the majority of the population who are impatient, yet want to create a wonderful life experience and will invest time and energy to do so.

The Short Course to Mental Wealth gets right to the essence of what is found in most self-help books. Anyone can use these powerful skills to making their life's experience joyous. John, paralyzed from the neck down did (p. 7); Morrie (*Tuesdays with Morrie*) stricken with Lou Gehrig's muscle-wasting disease did; so did Randy Pausch (*The Last Lecture*), terminal with pancreatic cancer. Many others have done so. Why not you?

We become our own genie in three phases:

1. becoming our own best friend

2. acquiring mental freedom from the prejudices of our nature and our nurturers

3. adding wisdom to our will to become a valuable member of the larger system to which

   we are an important part.

Why we need the wisdoms offered in *The Short Course to Mental Wealth*:

> *The unleashed power of the atom has changed everything save our modes of thinking and we thus drift toward unparalleled catastrophe ... a new type of thinking is essential if mankind is to survive and move toward higher levels.[2] .... The release of atomic energy has not created a new problem. It has merely made more urgent the necessity of solving an existing one.   Einstein*

Destructive aggression has been and continues to be our most universal problem. With the recent introduction and spread of powerful weapons to which there is no defense, we have become our own worst enemy. *The Short Course* introduces the **newer way of thinking** we require if we choose to transform our present *age of speed and greed* into one of *wise creeds and good deeds*. Educating our mind to become a powerful weapon for mass construction is our best hope to complete the road to civilization that we have thus far partially created. New technology enables us to rapidly spread mental wealth. I recommend starting with *The Short Course* because it will motivate you to continue on to the even more important book. The challenging full course, *A Newer Way of Thinking*, is for those who aspire to become the architects and engineers needed to complete the road to civility and world peace. It[3] explains <u>why</u> we remain stuck in a *partially civilized* state and <u>how</u> we may proceed to create the Nirvana we desire.

[2] The New York Times, May 25, 1946

[3] Especially the section *Good Aggression*

The preliminary step to becoming the genie that can make life's experience more wonderful is to become one's own best friend. *The Short Course* condenses the self-endorsement skills common to most personal growth books into an easily mastered no-nonsense curriculum. Genies must be freed before they grant wishes. Self-endorsement skills transform us from "love junkies" enslaved to others for our daily requirement of self-worth to become the powerful genie that can make our wishes for a fulfilling life a reality. Our freed personal genie is our means to use our best to do our best. We free our will from uncritical obedience to *what has been* and *what is* (instinct and habit) so that we may act with independence and originality (reason and wisdom) to create *what can be.* Becoming our marvelous lifelong traveling companion is among the most pleasurable of life's tasks.

Becoming our own best friend enables us to become potent lovers. Our gift of love to others will no longer be conditioned on what comes back; it becomes a joyous act complete in itself. Self-endorsement guarantees us immediate satisfaction from our own action, from what we do more than what others do. We are able to love our neighbor to the degree we learn the skill of loving our self. Skill in creating love enables us to become a citizen of the world, a valuable member of the greater community of which we are a member. Mature thinking allows us to add love to our communal wealth rather than only take, as we first are required. **Self-endorsement skills are also the source of patience.** The ability to reward our self now for work whose major benefits are not realized until some future time enables us to postpone immediate physical gratification for our greater long-term good.

Following the strens that emphasize the joyous task of learning to love our neighbor as our self, *The Short Course* introduces three original mental skills that go beyond our vast personal growth literature. In combination, they create a newer way of thinking that leads to *geniehood*. **(1) Seven substitutions to our vocabulary** free our will from the prejudices each of us inherit through our genes and acquire from our nurturers during our prolonged period of dependence. Thereafter, **(2) The Mental Response Control Panel** identifies the limited choices available to our freed will to process data into action. The *magical problem-solving sent*ence replaces the habitual negative choices including the two most common alternatives: the primitive responses of blaming others or our self, "guilting." Upon becoming our own best friend and freeing our will from its early masters, we may concentrate on **(3)** the **collection of strens** others have shown work, and those we newly create to expand our collective mental wealth.

We all want to *feel good* and *do good*! (Well, most everyone; I've met a few individuals who seem to enjoy being miserable.) If you are reading this *Short Course* I know you can create a wonderful life experience. Here is how I have proven this to myself. I would like to fly like a bird. I don't try anymore because I have never seen anyone flap their arms and get off the ground. However, if I saw just one person flapping their arms and flying, I'd become very excited and get at it. You see, I wouldn't need to see all people flying, not even a few; just one would be quite convincing. Now I have seen not just one but many individuals who *feel good* and *do good*! Some who really "make it" have the worst life situations imaginable, yet they have acquired the skills to *feel good* and *do good*; they created mental wealth! Likely, you have met or know of such individuals. I concluded if others could, I could. I did and so can you!

The Short Course was conceived when my son, a medical doctor, asked me if I could provide a simpler version to offer to his patients. I thought it a great idea and opportunity. Why not make the basic skills of *feeling good* and *doing good* easily available in professional offices and work places in addition to the Internet? The abbreviated version is designed to be studied in eight sections, each of about 10 pages. In my son's office, patients are provided copies of a few basic skills to get started applying the skills and experience the benefits. Successive skill-building sections are available on request. However, individuals are encouraged to continue *The Short Course* on their computer screen or print sections to study at a convenient time and place. Other sponsors may choose a different format to offer the course. In addition to *The Short Course*, the Internet site **www.anwot.org** contains the advanced course, *A Newer Way of Thinking*. The advanced course explains why we need to change our manner of thinking and emphasizes how our collective efforts will make a difference. The Internet books are both free.

You will learn that if you're like most people, **the way you think** is the main source of life's joy <u>and</u> misery! This is wonderful, wonderful news!

☺   If the manner we think is the major cause of *feeling good* and *doing good*, or its lack, we are in the best position to change. We have the power to educate ourselves; we have limited power to change "others" and/or the world. Mental skill-building is within our own control!

☺   The newer way of thinking to *feel good* and *do good* is "newer," <u>not</u> "new." We don't require learning a foreign language. The mental skills provided, along with the easy substitutions of the few *word-switches* within our native language are so simple, easily taught, and readily learned that most will understandably be skeptical.

The ANWOT curriculum to *feeling good* and *doing good* has five components:

▶ **1. Self-endorsement** (love-creation): **The Short Course** begins with directions on the mental skills we need to apply to become our own best friend. These exercises turn around the manner of thinking that is the source of becoming our own worst enemy. We live with *ourselves* 100% of the time, far more than the measly minutes we are engaged with others. Many persons go through life remaining "love junkies." They require that others provide their minimum daily requirement of self-worth instead of assuming responsibility for what they as adults can best do for themselves. As we acquire the skills of becoming our own best friend, our skill in abundant love-creation will spill-over. We experience the joy of giving to others.

Example: We provide vitamins and exercise for our body. Self-endorsements are the vitamins and exercise that keep our mind healthy. When you are thinking or look into a mirror, do you provide your mind its minimum daily requirement of endorsements? "I'm such a hot sketch." "Congratulations for doing my reasonable best!" *or* are you more likely to put in a few toxins? Do you recognize any self putdowns? Do you "should" on yourself?

▶ **2. Becoming our own person** (also referred to as *self*-mastery, *thought control*, and *mental freedom*): Next, we need to learn three easy word substitutions or *word-switches* that free our will from the demands and prejudices that our genes and nurturers inscribe into every native language. For many years *will* power is a slave to what others demand. These simple word-switches upgrade our manner of thinking from dependency and blind obedience to create our personal genie, to *become our own person* and the *director* and *producer* of our life's experience.

Example: A *word-switch* may be likened to the switch on a train track. A simple alteration at one point dramatically alters the path and outcome of action. **Prescriptive** *should* (*have to, must*) words demand that our thinking must obey authority according to the perspective of some "other." Substituting a **descriptive** *could* (*prefer, I am wise when ...*) word prompts the mind to consider problem-solving alternatives and assume personal choice-making responsibility. Updating the manner of thinking habitually practiced through our prolonged dependency requires only a few more appropriate word-switches to take control of our will power.

▶ **3. The Mental Response Control Panel**: Having acquired the mental skills of becoming our own best friend and freeing our will power from the prejudices of what we inherit and have been force fed, the Mental Response Control Panel explains the eight choices our will has available to direct mental energy to action. Two of these choices consistently lead to constructive outcomes; they work *for* us. Once we can recognize (label) them, we may consistently substitute the *problem–solving* and *self-endorsement* mental responses for the *blaming* responses and those others that are commonly a source of our problems.

Example: The most common harmful responses are primitive and easy to recognize – *Someone did what they shouldn't have done* or *someone didn't do what they should*. They lead to blaming others and/or "guilting" our self. We redirect our energy when we teach ourselves to instead think – *Given this situation, what's most likely to get me what I want, for me and you (us and them), for now and later. Congratulations to me for using reason and wisdom rather than instinct and habit.* With practice, the use of *problem-solving thinking* will become reduced from a sentence to a word and then become automatic and effortless, and those terrorists that presently dwell in our mind gradually wither away from lack of use.

▶ **4. Wisdom: A freed *Will* produces both *love* and *hate* until wisdom is added to power!** As we acquire the skills to become our own best friend, free our *will* from blind obedience to "others," and regularly apply the problem-solving skills that consistently work *for* us, we become motivated to collect the wisdoms others have made available to us. Wisdom allows us to *constructively* direct our energy to problem-solving rather than engage in *blaming others, guilting our self, worrying*, and the other alternatives that get us what we don't want.

Example: Teaching our *self* the skill of self-endorsement is one of the wisest uses of our will power. Wisdom gets a huge boost when we update our thinking with a few *word-switches* (as in 2.) and consistently apply *the problem-solving sentence*. The "strength stren" (page 7) is also a marvelous beginning to the collection of wisdoms provided in these pages and the growing collection available *free* on the Internet at **www.anwot.org** . We become more powerful genies as we acquire skill in selecting and creating the wisdoms that work best for us.

▶ **5. Values**: Mental freedom enables us to experience the joy of creating and owning the values that guide our life's work. Wisely begin with the two that have attained universal agreement among philosophers and our major religions:

A. *Love our neighbor as our self.* [Do you see why it is important to start with the self-endorsement skills to *become our own best friend*?]

B. The Golden Rule: *Treat others as we would have them treat us.* [When, due to our new self-endorsement skills, we can enjoy but no longer require others to provide our daily requirement of self-worth, we experience the joy of unconditionally offering our growing mental wealth to others.]

Use of this educational course to *feeling good* and *doing good*:

Consider this ***Short Course to Mental Wealth*** as the continuation of our formal primary education, which, for most, stopped before age eighteen, just about the time our mind reaches optimum maturity to pursue a graduate degree in **Feeling Good** and **Doing Good**.

These skills enable us to become Chief Executive Officer of our life's direction, assume control of what we will produce in our lifetime and how we participate in the larger system to which we are a part. Let's free our will, add wisdom, and become the genie that makes our prayers come true.

Mastery of the *3 R's* that we learned in grade school required study and practice over time; a book to be simply read as a novel would not do. Similarly, success in the process of *becoming our own person* as we free our will from the prejudices of instinct and our nurturers may be likened to learning to walk, playing a musical instrument or becoming skilled in a profession. **Skill is acquired through repetition!** In every skill-building process, repetition of the basics is required while gradually increasing competence. Some best learn with lots of repetition. A graduate degree certifies competence in a number of individual skills, *each* acquired through multiple repetitions as we proceed to more advanced levels. If impatience and/or boredom sets in with mastery of the simpler skills, rapidly skim or skip over the duplication no longer needed. Building mental strength is a joyous lifetime endeavor!

The road to *self*-mastery began for you, me, and all of us as mental slaves to what nature and our nurturers first make of us. Mental freedom is acquired step-by-step. Work on one or two strens before going on to the next. Excellence is built on knowledge and application. Although we can expect immediate benefits, *feeling good* and *doing good* grow as we increase our collection of strens. Graciously accept the mistakes that skill-building requires. Periodic review of first skills will add new insights made apparent only upon familiarity with more advanced skills. Recall that *mental muscles*, like physical muscles, work best when individual strands work together. The wisdom of the group is greater than the sum of its individual units.

Participation in a discussion group and/or sharing strens with others boosts learning and increases our satisfaction. Share portions or this entire guide. Use its contents as you wish, when you wish, with no obligation on your part, save one requirement -- if any material is to be used for profit, prior authorization is required. Please help popularize ANWOT by acquiring the skills and becoming a role model to inspire others. You are invited to make copies of **The Short Course**; adding your own strens makes a nice personalized gift.

Each one, teach one!

1. The *Strength* Stren

This stren is one of the most powerful wisdoms. It is literally "the strength" stren. I acquired it from an individual who overcame the most devastating of life's circumstances.

John is a paraplegic. His broken neck changed his life when he was a teen. It was a game of football turned tragedy. From that day, he no longer had control of his legs or arms. Physically he knew he would be dependent on others for whatever time he would live. Yet, when I met John, he was applying for a job as a senior therapist. A helper took him to classes and literally turned the pages. He earned his doctorate in psychology. He met a woman with shared interests and they married. He and his wife were raising their adopted daughter. He was not simply alive; he was living and loving his life.

How had he turned himself around? What made the difference? I had to ask and I'm so glad I did for I received the gift of this stren, which I can now pass on to you. Here is his response, as close as I can remember:

"For several years I was miserable. My thoughts were constant that I didn't want to live. And then one day I had the thought that changed my life:

As long as I thought about what I'd lost, what I didn't have, or might not attain, I realized I would continue to feel miserable. I began to focus my attention on what I had attained, what I had available to me right now, and what I might yet attain. This simple idea changed everything."

Too often, too many people dwell on what they have lost, what they don't have now, and/or what they may never obtain. This is the sure formula to create misery. I have sent this stren to friends at holiday time and received many grateful comments to verify its effectiveness. My most recent letter was from a young woman whose father died recently; she turned her thoughts and feelings around when she began to focus on her happy experiences with her dad and all she had received.

"There were two prisoners looking through the bars;
the one saw mud, the other saw stars." Anon.

When we experience any loss, one of the many of life's unfairness and/or setbacks, it is normal to hurt. Why unnecessarily add to the necessary hurt by dwelling on the loss, guilt, or the missing part of our life? Who would go to the supermarket, pay for their food, and then get back in line to pay for the food again? It's hard enough to have to deal with the loss; why compound it? Though it may take time and not be easy, we <u>do</u> have the resources to get over the blows fate deals us. Keep this in mind and stop the negative nonproductive mental dwelling!

SECTION ONE ▮

2. THIS STREN[4] DEALS WITH SELF-ENDORSEMENT

We are, by nature's design, prone to distort events toward the negative; there is no corresponding inherited tendency to think optimistically. The earliest function of conscious awareness (consciousness), in animals and humans, is to protect us from danger, to survive by anticipating what we lack and any source of harm. Our primitive innate consciousness has programmed us from birth to seek what we need and to avoid what is dangerous. This has been identified as our inherited "fight or flight" response.

The concerns of early thoughts are generally physical such as food, warmth, and other biologic needs that provide for our life and safety. These innate patterns for self-preservation direct us to focus on "the empty part of the glass" and tend towards worry because it has survival value. We preoccupy ourselves with the aggressors that may cause harm. We are prone to get stuck in such negative thinking. Animals are not known for laughter, and I have read that primitive humankind did not laugh at all. In evolution, humor is a relatively recent human invention that many contemporaries scarcely engage in. Ditto for "optimism." How often have you heard someone say "I've spent the night worrying" (anticipating the worst) as compared to "I spent the night optimizing" (anticipating the best)?

In addition, and perhaps of greater importance, the means we are taught to be "civilized" and curb physical aggression ("you shouldn't fight") is to become *mentally* aggressive. We acquire skill in blaming, dominating, winning, being "right," competing, wanting, and surviving using mental means. We are expected to "succeed" at a high level. When we don't meet the expectations of "others," be as good or nice as we "should," we quite skillfully verbally attack ourselves. This human invention is called "guilt." We demean and criticize ourselves. In my observation, we commonly become "our own worst enemy." We attack ourselves with words and thoughts, make ourselves depressed, and may even physically attack ourselves. In the extreme, we call this "murdering oneself" or suicide. We engage in self-putdowns like no other creature. Perfectionists tend to make themselves especially miserable while most develop advanced skills in self-blame. The expected and observed outcome is anxiety, worry, depression, apathy, and related attributes of a difficult life experience.

[4] Stren – any idea, bit of wisdom, attitude, feeling, experience, behavior, or mental skill that strengthens well-being.

For these reasons, we are wise to teach our *self* the skill of calling forth both positive thinking and positive feelings. This easy to learn mental skill is called "Self-endorsement." The highest level of our adult brain (the cortex) is sufficiently complex and sophisticated that we can attain a level of joy and well-being not available to other creatures. Rather than remaining dominated by our innate, automatic pessimism, and the acquired thinking patterns of blaming others and ourselves, we are capable of developing our own personal, creative, problem-solving patterns. Through human creativity, most persons reading this stren (you included) have already gone beyond attending to their (your) immediate physical needs.

Mature human consciousness is not dominated by the survival needs of the physical self. Rather than being limited to focusing on the immediate moment, we may scan time, past/present/future, and deal with reality through mental rehearsal (thinking).

Our human consciousness may readily be taught to recognize past positive accomplishments, present achievements and acquisitions, and goals yet to come, so that we may generate appreciation and positive feelings now. The ability to keep the positive in focus and not to simply dwell on the negative, on what is missing in our life, is a basic skill for maintaining positive feelings. To make misery, simply dwell on what you have lost, don't have now, or may not get. Teach yourself to focus on what you have achieved, have now, and can yet accomplish. Wow! That is the wise choice available to each of us.

Self-endorsement is the process by which we can teach our *self* to become our own best friend and remove the natural distortion created by a primitive consciousness whose function is primarily designed to focus on what is missing. Our primitive thinking has limited capacity to dwell on what we've accomplished, what we have now, or what we can attain in the future. Self-appreciation, gratitude, and love are skills we hopefully have been fortunate enough to have been taught by our nurturers. More productively, we may now teach our *self*.

In sum, worry and negative anticipation are strongly biologic. To what nature provides, we soon acquire skill in habitually directing aggression inward, in blaming and demeaning ourselves. Self-endorsement will remain in its natural feeble state until we nourish it to dominance. The conversation we engage in within, too often, is our major source of unhappiness. The characters that carry on a dialogue within our thoughts and thinking will remain poor lifetime traveling companions unless we develop the skill of self-endorsement. Our effort is one of the best investments we can make. We can develop both intellectual (knowing) endorsement and emotional (feeling) endorsement skills. Together, they work great.

There are many ways to grow your skill in self-endorsement, to become our own best friend:

Make a list of all the important positives you have. Review your positives regularly so that you can easily call them to your awareness. Whenever you identify a new positive, add it to the list; make it grow! Remind these positives to yourself frequently throughout the day, especially when you think of your favorite putdowns and/or worries, and until habit effortlessly replaces your no-longer-needed written list.   Watch out for "yes buts." Consider this example of positives offered by one person who made it work:

☺ I have life.

☺ I have the capacity to think, to teach myself, to grow, to fulfill myself.

☺ I have the ability to smile, laugh, and feel good and inflation doesn't raise the price of a laugh.

☺ I recognize others who have far less health, wealth, or opportunity than I, yet they seem genuinely to enjoy themselves, and living. That others can, I know there is a way!!!

☺ I have the capacity to engage regularly in interesting dialogue with myself and with others.

☺ I have reasonable security from physical harm.

☺ I live at a time and place in the world where I have better than ever opportunities for personal freedom, health, education, travel, work, and physical comforts.

☺ Important parts of me work well: my ability to learn, my vital organs, and most everything else.

☺ I have people in my life who love me or would help me. These people include my wife, my children, family, my family of friends, and a number of people I can develop as support people.

☺ I have people in my life that can enjoy what I have to offer - family, friends, and humanity.

☺ Even if I reach a place in my life where I don't know anyone, there are fellow humans who are more than willing to help (clergy, professional counselors, or lay persons who are self-sufficient or supported by the community). My government is available to offer me care if I need it and when I ask for it.

☺ I possess the skill of reading, writing, talking, and I could go on quite a bit here.

☺ I have work skills such as conscientiousness, expressiveness, formal education, and I could add many more here. I am capable of teaching myself new skills, and there are vast human and material resources available to me, free for the taking.

☺ I have made the following accomplishment: I like myself, have good friends, have developed adaptation skills, and I can add many more.

☺ Positive qualities others have told me about myself include warmth, patience, empathy, an interest in people, and a number of others I could identify.

☺ Positive qualities I have include the willingness to work, to love, to laugh at my mistakes, and many other qualities I could identify.

☺ What I lack that is really important, including becoming a good friend to myself, I can attain.

Personally, I find it helpful to remind myself that I, and most of us, live better today than the kings of recent times. We have a healthier and better selection of foods; libraries, mass media, and technology that provide educational opportunity; greater comforts in our home, work, and environment; a more welcoming bed (ah!); unprecedented sanitation, medical and surgical means to improve the quality and quantity of life; and so much more could be said.

The Bookshelf: In your mind, create a bookshelf loaded with books. In distinct print, put a label on as many books as you can, identifying some experience, topic, interest, fantasy, event, etc. that you like to think about. Some of these examples may get you started: My Favorite Person; Music I like; My Collection of Fun Times; Funny Stories; When I Win the Lottery; What I Believe (religious or otherwise); My Ideal Romantic Experience; The Perfect Beauty Appointment; Great Athletes; My Next Great Meal; Jobs I'd Enjoy; Great Sexual Pleasure; What Do I Want in Life?; Work I Enjoy Doing; Books That Got Me To Think; Where I'm Happiest; Dreams to Have Tonight; Hobbies That Interest Me; Good Things in Retirement, and so on. Keep your mental bookshelf in your mind's eye. Try to keep your book titles in sight. When you become aware you are dwelling on negative talk with yourself, first give yourself a pat on the back for recognizing the old patter. Then, pull one of your books off the shelf and get as thoroughly involved as you can. If you're like most, you'll find it gets easier with practice.

Challenging negative distortions:

Now comes the practical application of your resources to teach yourself to challenge your negatives and to experience feeling better and doing better in your life through self-endorsement. When people engage in negative thinking, they often totally overlook the greater number of positives in their lives. This creates a distortion. Most people distort habitually. Your written list of positives can serve as your resource to balance your negative thinking.

For daily practice: Write out some of your biggest negatives and current worries on paper to keep near your list of positives. Every time you spot a negative idea about your*self*, balance it with positives. With regular practice, this will become habitual and so automatic that it will require little effort. Once you start to realize the power and control you have over your feelings, you will find that you will practice tuning in to the positives even more frequently. You will develop your "thought control" muscles for feeling well in addition to doing well, and you will create increasingly growing fulfillment in your life. It's great to have your*self* as your best friend.

The Tape Recording: You have the ability to listen in on the conversation you carry on with yourself. Imagine you tape record this conversation several times throughout the day. When you play it back, how would you describe the dialogue? Does it sound like two good friends speaking with one another? Is there interesting dialogue? Can you detect enthusiasm? Or are there significant periods of criticisms, boredom, worry, blaming, self-pitying, and so on? Why not strive to change the quality of that internal conversation so that your taped segments become increasingly positive? Do it! Your efforts can make it work.

Follow *Self-endorsement* with the stren *"Emotional self-endorsement."* They dramatically strengthen the important skill -- PATIENCE.

----

3. THIS STREN DEALS WITH: EMOTIONAL SELF-ENDORSEMENT

Good feelings stir us to continued action. Immediate satisfaction is critical to sustain the work and practice required to attain the natural rewards of virtually every important skill, viz. getting an education, sustaining a relationship, keeping physically fit, playing a musical instrument, growing a garden, and growing our capacity for loving our *self* and others. Emotional endorsement is the main source of immediate satisfaction to enjoy the work we do now in order to attain more satisfaction later. Knowing we are doing something worthwhile is intellectual endorsement; its satisfaction is usually weaker than emotional joy. Joining emotional endorsement to intellectual endorsement provides the most effective incentive to continue our efforts.

How often have you known what you believed was wisest and preferred to do, but instead did what felt better right at that time? Get the idea? Understanding simply isn't enough!

Few persons know how to emotionally endorse themselves. We get little training in this skill. You know how to say to yourself, "I did a good job," or, "That was nice," but after you say those things you go right on to the next worry or problem to be solved. You don't extract all the honey you can from your efforts. Yet you are probably more than well-developed in the opposite of emotional *self*-endorsement, *self*-blame. When you became intellectually aware of a shortcoming, you experienced guilt, shame, or embarrassment within every fiber of your being. Most are so practiced at blaming-in that the negative feelings come automatically, seemingly without effort or intention. Could you imagine that you can teach yourself to create "feeling good" with the same ease that you "naturally" feel guilty, embarrassed, ashamed or depressed? You can! ... if you become aware of how to endorse yourself emotionally and practice doing so.

Since you know how to emotionally blame yourself, you already have the skills for emotional endorsement. The problem is that you direct your emotional endorsement to others. Think of the times you've expressed yourself in such a way as to stimulate a response from your [a] dog -- you know how to get that dog to wag its tail, shake its behind, and get thoroughly excited. You've probably called forth great enthusiasm in doing the same kind of thing with a child. You've even emotionally endorsed food. "Wow! Look at that fantastic, gooey ice cream creation!" Recall the enthusiasm with which you've applauded a great musical performance or cheered for your team at a sports event. You just haven't had much direction and experience in emotional *self*-endorsement, in "wowing" yourself. The skill is there. It simply needs to be directed to yourself. Most people are familiar with directing emotional blame to themselves, but unfortunately they were taught that it's "selfish" to emotionally endorse themselves. One man recalled being told, "Praise only counts if it comes from someone else." (This is one reason most of us become so dependent on what we imagine others might be thinking about us.)

When you do something worthwhile (i.e., your "reasonable best," which is virtually always in your control!!!), could you imagine a gala brass band marching down Main Street? Two people are carrying a banner that stretches across the whole street with streamers being tossed about and people are cheering you from their windows? There you are, smack in the middle of the parade, smiling proudly and waving, "Yep, I did it all right. It was me." Such a *self*-endorsement tool in your repertoire is much more likely to call forth your emotions than an intellectual, flat, "That was O.K." Use this image and/or create your own as a regular *self*-endorsement tool.

Some people can use or develop their existing creative imagery and fantasy to initiate enthusiasm. Others find it easier to call forth feelings of joy, inspiration, and enthusiasm from prior experiences. Make a mental scrapbook of times you've felt loved, got a pat on the shoulder, experienced joy, happiness, or enthusiasm. Permit yourself to call these "snapshots" forth to re-create similar good feelings. Combine past experience with the present creative imagery to develop the results you want.

Experiment by creating your own skills in emotional *self*-endorsement. Try it when you wake up in the morning. What do you say to yourself when you first look in the mirror? "What a hot sketch I am!" Or do you presently say something else? If you are like most people who are practiced in the art of emotionally *self*-blaming, but are weak in emotionally endorsing yourself, apply your conscious awareness to nurture *self*-endorsement. Your efforts will be amply rewarded. Practice! Practice! Practice!

Act as if

"Act as if" is another very effective method to change and/or create new emotions. Even if you have difficulty experiencing emotional *self*-endorsement, go through the motions. Imagine you had a part to play on the stage. As every actor knows, if you put yourself in the role and go through the motions, the "act as if" gradually becomes "feel as if" and then the "as if" weakens. A genuinely new sentiment is created. What successful actors need to learn, so you also can.

Remind yourself that the old put-me-downs ... "stupid," "jerk," "stupid jerk," "you don't deserve ...," "shame," "asshole," and so on [what is your favorite put-down word(s)?] call forth powerful emotions that have been thriving many years. Recognize that you are wise to get rid of the old "demons" so well learned in the past. Those put-downs now mostly serve as terrorists! In a sense, you'd be wise to kill them off; become a murderer to the useless baggage you carry with you. Yes, it's fun to vigorously attack these intruders ... and you hurt no one in so doing.

So here again, even though you feel the emotions attached to these old put-me-downs, act as if they don't belong, they are unwelcome! Take on the role of "good guy" getting rid of the demons, clean out the "bad," make room for the positive invited guests. Whether you are strengthening your "attaboy/attagirl" *self*-endorsing skill or attacking the put-me-downs, your use of the "act as if" technique can help your attitude to become more positive. However, I believe it is most productive to emphasize directing your energy to creating positive sentiment. The old demons will wither away if you stop feeding them with your attention and instead direct your energy to creating more muscles of *self*-endorsement.

[Note: Follow this stren with "Secondary Endorsement" -- it fits right in.]

SECONDARY ENDORSEMENT

Once you recognize the value of *self*-endorsement and begin to combine both intellectual and emotional *self*-endorsement, you can initiate the skill of creating good feelings as an effortless habit. Your task will become much easier if you also develop the skill of secondary endorsement. Endorse yourself for the very, very worthy act of endorsing yourself!

Your first experiences with generating emotional *self*-endorsement will be a bit like forging a path through the jungle. Unless regularly cultivated, the new path will soon be overgrown. Not even a trace of the hard-to-cut path will remain. The long established negligence in taking care of your emotional needs and/or *self* put-downs re-appear and will, predictably, soon overpower the new.

Self-endorsement provides immediate encouragement for constructive acts whose natural rewards may not come until far in the future. When you endorse yourself, you are engaging in one of the most constructive acts available to you. Therefore, give yourself credit each time you endorse yourself. "Hurrah! Congratulations to me for endorsing my *self*. That's worthy of a special bonus."

Secondary endorsement is the opposite of secondary blaming (blaming yourself when you realize you're still putting yourself down). By now, you may be wise enough to label instances of blaming-in, and soon stop putting yourself down when you make an error, when you "do what you shouldn't," or, "don't do what you should have." But since you, like most people, are a creature of habit, it will be only a matter of time before you recognize you are still blaming yourself. You say, "I'm so stupid; I should have learned that by now!" This "secondary blaming," i.e. blaming yourself for blaming yourself, is far more persistent than secondary endorsement. It's putting yourself down because you are aware that you are still putting yourself down and you "shouldn't do that!" Once you recognize this tendency of, as one person described, "shoulding" on yourself, yourself-putdowns will become apparent like a blinking light bulb. "Pull-ups," i.e. *self*-endorsements, serve you better than putdowns.

Just as secondary blaming is a variation of blaming yourself, secondary endorsement is a special variation of *self*-endorsement. Instead of pulling yourself down with each act of blaming-in, when you endorse yourself for endorsing yourself, you pull yourself up and keep yourself up. Teach yourself to become consciously aware of any endorsement you initiate when you do something worthwhile. As soon as you recognize that you're endorsing yourself, call forth images such as blinking lights, musical accolades, and cheers as your signal to automatically trigger the secondary endorsement you deserve for endorsing yourself. This reinforcement can escalate the intensity of the immediate pleasure you experience and create the energy you need to overcome your old, established, negative patterns. Once the patterns of blaming, avoidance, worry, and helplessness/hopelessness are established within you, they cling tenaciously until you substitute the positive pattern of *self*-endorsement.

Practice: Endorse yourself again each time you catch yourself endorsing yourself.

----

4. <u>YOU NEED EMOTIONAL MDRs, TOO</u>

This stren deals with your minimum daily requirement [MDR] for approval.

Caroline was having an especially difficult day. Before she left for work, her husband complained that she never showed any interest in his career. At the office, her boss rejected the proposal she'd put extra effort into, and her secretary quit, telling her she was impossible to work for. Caroline sat at her desk, took a deep breath, and closed her eyes. She pictured herself marching down Main Street, the VIP in a parade. A brass band playing, "The Most Beautiful Girl in the World," marched behind her. Two young women dressed in colorful costumes walked along in front of her, carrying a banner that stretched across the street. The banner read, "Hurrah for Caroline!"

After a few minutes of engaging in her "pick me up" fantasy, Caroline returned to reality with renewed energy and enthusiasm. She took problem-solving action. She put in a requisition for another secretary, phoned her husband saying she wanted to discuss his complaint, and began revising her proposal.

Six months ago, if Caroline were confronted with only one of the circumstances she found herself in, she would have dwelled on her shortcomings, mentally beat on herself, become depressed, and considered herself a failure. Now, she is able to look at criticisms from others objectively, without putting herself down.

Caroline came to see me because of her recurring bouts of depression and a variety of physical complaints, including headache, stomach queasiness, and insomnia. I soon discovered that Caroline's depression was usually dependent on others' reactions to her. If people praised her or otherwise showed their approval, she felt good about herself and remained in a cheerful frame of mind. She seemed unable to cope with critical comments, however. Whether or not the criticisms were valid wasn't the issue. Because she didn't possess the skill of providing for her self-esteem, Caroline reacted to the criticism with a depression that was often incapacitating, causing her to stay in bed or lie down with a headache.

Caroline was an intelligent young woman who was well informed about physical fitness and nutrition. She obtained at least the MDR (minimum daily requirement) of her physical needs, such as vitamins and minerals. It appeared to me that she pampered her flesh, but neglected and even abused her mental well-being. One day, I asked her if she paid any attention to <u>emotional</u> MDRs.

"No," she smiled weakly. "I've never heard of such a thing."

"Could you imagine that just as your body has minimum needs for certain physical substances, your emotions also have daily requirements?"

"I'm not sure what you're getting at."

"I'm saying that you can feel better about yourself and suffer far less from depression by taking responsibility for giving yourself your MDRs of emotional nutrition."

"What do you mean by MDRs of emotional nutrition?"

"Your emotional MDR is the minimum daily requirement of positive feelings about yourself that you need each day to sustain your well-being."

"How can I give these MDRs to myself?"

"By substituting positive statements for the negative, demoralizing statements you usually make about yourself. Look in the mirror first thing in the morning and tell yourself, 'I'm lovable. I'm a hot sketch.' Or sing about your accomplishments while you're in the shower, walk proud, as if you know you're somebody. Recognize and let go of self-pity, blaming, and 'what-if' worrying; use your newfound energy to develop an attitude of gratitude. Assign yourself a unit every time you think or say something positive about yourself until you reach, let's say, at least ten a day. You can add up the units in a notebook or just do it mentally."

Caroline was skeptical, but she agreed to try what I suggested. Like many depressed individuals, at first she had difficulty thinking of anything positive to say about her *self*. With a bit of effort, however, she began to list some qualities that led her to believe that she was just as worthwhile as anyone else. She decided, for instance, that she was friendly, neat, and a hard worker. By focusing her attention on what she had, her accomplishments, and what she might attain, she had less time to put her*self* down. Her mood improved. One day, she decided to jot down the units of approval she received from others. At the end of the day, her total was two. "If I depended on others for my emotional MDRs, I'd be depressed most of the time," she said.

Caroline, like most of us, was far too dependent on what others thought of her. She let her mood be controlled by people and events that were, predictably, unpredictable. It was appropriate for Caroline and for all of us to depend on others for our emotional MDRs when we were children. Children don't have the mental resources to create their own feelings of self-worth. As adults, we don't have to continue to react in the same way; indeed, we are unwise to remain so dependent.

We are encouraged to do more and more for ourselves as we continue to mature. We dress ourselves, take care of our personal needs, decide on our lifestyle, and learn to support ourselves. In virtually every area of life, we are taught, and expected, to take care of ourselves, <u>except</u> insofar as our emotional well-being is concerned.

Wouldn't you be insulted if, at this stage of your life, someone tried to brush your teeth for you or feed you? Yet with respect to your emotional needs, not only are you not taught to provide for your well-being, but you are even taught not to be kind to yourself. You are admonished if you say good things about yourself, especially if you share your self-satisfaction with others.

Larry, an engineer with an interest in photography, was pleased with the darkroom he had just built. He took a great deal of pride in showing it to his friends. One evening, his mother took him aside and told him he was acting like a braggart. "She always told me that praise only counts if it comes from someone else. She says I'm selfish, vain, and an egotist if I say anything good about myself or what I've done."

Larry had worked hard at providing for his emotional MDRs. His darkroom was near the top of his list. Larry's mother didn't recognize that he was simply attempting to share his accomplishments with others, not lord it over them.

We are so strongly taught not to provide for our emotional MDRs that most people find it very difficult to do so. We understand that it's healthy to use our energy for self-encouragement rather than self-blame. Yet the lifelong repetition of self-putdowns such as, "I'm stupid," "I'm a jerk," or, "I should've known!" are so ingrained and so natural, that making positive statements about our self feels awkward. Don't become discouraged if you don't get immediate results with your emotional MDRs. Think of the units of self-put-downs you've been giving yourself daily. With lots of practice, the way you would gradually tone up a muscle, the positive statements can catch up with, challenge, and overtake your habitual, negative put-downs.

Just as we don't know the exact number of vitamins, minerals, amino acids, and other requirements we need to enjoy optimum physical health, we don't know the exact number of MDRs we need to satisfy our emotional well-being. As we increasingly create more of our emotional MDRs, however, we'll sustain our well-being more confidently.

As you experiment with this idea, you'll discover the number of MDRs you need to give you "fuel" to carry you through the day. Ten units was Caroline's starting point. You can also start with ten and increase the amount up to twenty, thirty, or many more units daily. You'll know that you have created sufficient MDRs when you're able to maintain your well-being on a consistent basis, and face life's challenges both energetically and enthusiastically.

Taking responsibility for our self-esteem doesn't imply that it's inappropriate to welcome and enjoy the approval of others. Approval, recognition, love, and support are worth working for. But when we take responsibility for our own emotional MDRs, what we get from others becomes a bonus, rather than a necessity. And you'll find that when you're less needy, it is easier to be a lover than a love "junky."

Take time each day to provide for both your physical and your emotional well-being. After you exercise, or while you're eating breakfast, take a few moments to consider your emotional MDRs. You can give yourself MDRs anytime and anyplace, but if you become accustomed to doing so at certain times of the day, you will form the habit quickly. Make a short, positive statement to yourself; "Attagirl!" ["Attaboy!"] Or use detailed imagery, such as the brass band fantasy Caroline engaged in.

As you begin to feel consistently good about yourself, you'll notice that people will enjoy being with you and seek out your company more often. People are attracted to a person with an upbeat attitude. The friends and popularity everyone desires are far more likely to develop when you no longer need others to reassure you that you're O.K. And you can add your new, upbeat attitude to your list of emotional MDRs.

SECTION TWO █

5. THE REASONABLE BEST MEASURE OF *SELF*-WORTH

This stren explains an appropriate measure of your actions that maintains *self*-worth.

One of the most effective and consistent ways to feel good about yourself is to apply the *reasonable best* stren. By recognizing when you're doing your reasonable best in a situation and giving yourself credit for doing so, you can create and maintain positive feelings about yourself.

What is the reasonable best test?

Most people evaluate their self-worth by the "outcome" of what they do. The reasonable best stren is an "input" measure of *self*-worth, that is, it emphasizes your efforts, not the results of your efforts.

In every situation in which you're trying to achieve a goal, you only have control of your input. The outcome is usually influenced by many factors that you can do little or nothing about. Unless you're a magician, you're unrealistic to expect that you can control the outcome of what you or others do. Yet most people have been taught since childhood to regulate their feelings about themselves by asking themselves the inappropriate outcome question, "Did it work out O.K.?" As a child, you didn't have the mental resources to apply the reasonable best stren. You had no choice but to be dependent on others for your *self*-worth.

Do you still depend on the outcome of your efforts as the primary measure of your *self*-worth? Consider these outcome measures that create a positive or negative feeling response:

I'm OK if:

I won.	The audience applauds.
My efforts worked out.	You understand.
They accept me.	They think I'm attractive.
I got an "A."	I own a ----------.
He/she loves me.	The kids do well.
My salary is increased.	I didn't make a mistake.

You're utilizing healthy, realistic criteria to create positive feelings about yourself whenever you answer, "Yes," to the question, "Am I doing my reasonable best?" even if you don't attain the outcome you desire! Yes, there may be necessary hurt and trauma because of the outcome. Almost always, we can't control the consequences of events; we can control how we deal with them. We worsen and sustain the effect of an undesired outcome by attacking our *self*-esteem. We often become our own worst enemy. (The above is worthwhile reviewing a number of times; what follows may help clarify the key aspects of the reasonable best stren.)

<u>But isn't it only natural to feel bad when things don't work out?</u>

Of course. Most people would be disappointed, sad, or hurt when the outcome of their efforts doesn't work out the way they had hoped. Maybe you didn't get that raise. In fact, you just lost your job after twenty years with the same company. Or you recently discovered that your son is involved with drugs and is "hanging out" with friends that you consider undesirable. Or you didn't get back the love you so desired from that special someone.

It's appropriate to experience discomfort and diminution of your spirits when things don't work out the way you would have liked, or when you've been treated unfairly. These feelings are normal and healthy, but you are designed to stand the hurt that comes when "the world doesn't cooperate." Applying the reasonable best stren balances your pain or disappointment. By creating a sustained level of positive feelings about your*self*, you become confident that you can manage your discomfort while facing the issues and attempting to resolve them.

<u>How do I know what my reasonable best is?</u>

Your reasonable best is the best you can do in a situation considering your limited resources. Your intelligence is far from perfect. You have restrictions of time and commitments to other obligations. Note that your reasonable best isn't your absolute best. For instance, suppose you want to win the annual bonus at work for obtaining the largest number of new accounts. You work at achieving this goal eighteen hours a day, seven days a week for several months. In this situation, you are doing your absolute best at the expense, by the way, of your spouse, children, friends, and even your health. This is more than most rational people would expect of you and it's more than is wise for you to expect of your*self*.

If you're in doubt about what your reasonable best is, discuss your efforts and expectations with other people. Seek the views of others to enhance your own critical appraisal. Others' opinions may be helpful in shedding light on your blind spots. Some people, characteristically perfectionists, set such unrealistically high standards for themselves that they think they are never doing enough. They continually feel inadequate, even though they do far more than their reasonable best. Others feel good about their *self* although they put forth little effort and accomplish almost nothing. Discussing with others what you believe is your reasonable best can provide valuable guidelines for your use in setting realistic goals.

<u>Suppose I'm not doing my reasonable best? Don't I deserve to feel bad about myself?</u>

Certainly not. You'll always be less than perfect at doing your reasonable best.
Improvement requires practice and patience; setbacks are to be expected along the way.

Each time you recognize you aren't doing your reasonable best, you create an
opportunity to improve in your endeavors until you reach the level of your reasonable best.
Your appropriate response is to say,
> "I didn't do my reasonable best, but I'm recognizing the fact that I could be doing
> better. Only by recognizing an imperfection can I take the positive step of calling
> forth more effort and teaching my *self* to do better. I deserve to feel good about
> my *self* for facing my shortcoming." (Most people beat on themselves when they
> discover they aren't the way they "should" be. Such *self*-putdowns lead to avoiding
> facing faults).

**Becoming aware of shortcomings, imperfections, or mistakes is your reasonable
best! It is one of the most productive things you can do because it affords you the
opportunity to discover a better way.** The reasonable best measure of *self*-worth prepares
us to apply problem-solving and learn from each of our mistakes.

There is no benefit to putting our *self* down because we are less than perfect, less
than we would desire to be. This is a negative response that uses our valuable energy
without correcting the situation. The most miserable persons I know are often perfectionists.
As it is, **the mistakes we make or our occasional poor judgment will probably lead to
unpleasant consequences. Why unnecessarily pay twice by attacking our *self*-worth?**
Once we pay for something, is it wise to keep going back to pay again and again?

Applying the reasonable best stren as a measure of *self*-worth may feel awkward at
first, just as mastering any new skill would. Learning to walk, talk, write, or play a musical
instrument all require practice. Merely understanding the reasonable best stren won't
provide you with good feelings about yourself. You'll need lots of practice to become
adept at using this input measure of *self*-worth. How often and how long have you been
practicing being controlled by the outcome of your actions?

Make the *reasonable best* stren a habit by asking yourself frequently during the day, "Am I
doing what I reasonably can?" If the answer is "yes," immediate, enthusiastic self-endorsement
(see stren "Emotional self-endorsement") is in order. If the answer is "no," congratulate
yourself for finding an opportunity to improve in your efforts. Ask yourself what you can
do to act more wisely now or in the future. Turn the answer to the question, "Am I doing my
reasonable best?" into a *self*-endorsing, problem-solving response. Whether the answer is "yes"
or "no," you will have created a win-win situation for growth and *self*-worth.

As you gain proficiency in this stren, you'll gradually free yourself from depending
on others or on random circumstances to maintain your *self*-worth. You'll consistently feel
good about your*self* because you can learn to do your reasonable best virtually 100% of the
time.

6. <u>FORGIVENESS</u>

This stren is my attempt to explain why *forgiveness* is one of (or) the most powerful of mental skills to increase peace of mind and peace in the world.

"Forgive them, for they know not what they do." Perhaps these are among the most important words ever spoken. Forgiveness = for + giving. I tend to equate forgiveness with love. Love is action that adds a positive experience to the world. It is a gift of our own creation for an "other" and/or our *self* to enjoy. I believe forgiveness is primarily a human quality because we create it using our unique language-equipped cortical brain. For the same reason, we are also distinguished by the degree we engage in hatred, prejudice, resentment, blaming others and ourselves (guilt). Please consider my explanation of the validity of this insight.

Destructive aggression is a basic means earth's creatures, us included, sustain the life cycle, establish a territory, obtain food, reproduce, and protect their young. We inherently act to serve our *self* and those we identify as "our family," often at the expense of others. *I* (and we) am (are) prepared to deal with *not I* and *them* with little regard for their well-being. Imagine how our gene's message would be expressed in words:

> *The world is for your benefit, to provide your needs and wants. Seek immediate pleasure; avoid immediate pain. If it feels good, tastes good, looks good, sounds good, take it if you can. Have little regard for the well-being of what's not me (us).*

Nature's way, *survival of the fittest*, as discussed elsewhere in the <u>Guide</u>, is not a strong supporter of forgiveness. Quite the opposite! It may better be described as an advocate of "fortakeness" = for + taking. The power to dominate others is basic to obtain one's needs. Nature's way is essentially amoral, self-centered, impatient, and an advocate of destructive (and constructive) aggression.

With the last to develop portion of the brain, the cortex, we acquire the ability to create symbols, store them, manipulate them to form ideas and concepts, and to effect physical change in the common world we share. This is a somewhat "magical" feat. Think about it. We represent physical reality in our mind by nonphysical concepts and ideas, manipulate these symbols to originate new perspectives, and then, generate will power sufficient to initiate what was not previously present in the common physical reality we share. If an individual were to show us an empty hat, cover it, and then pull out a rabbit, we may call that person a magician. With symbols, our mind is regularly performing such magical acts: physical → mental → will power → physical

The "magic" within our cortex to transform physical reality into concepts, ideas, and the like using symbols to create virtual or nonphysical reality is what we call consciousness. The reverse process, whereby we apply our virtual personal reality to make a difference in the common reality is what we call will power. We can understand that this magical ability of our complex brain requires considerable time to mature; and the degree of magical power will depend not only on the capacity of the cortex but also on the quality of the symbols with which it has to work. Some thinking programs are more sophisticated than others and of course one's native language may have been designed to emphasize a limited perspective.

I believe the truth of the matter is that the earliest programming of consciousness is dominated by our genes survival of the fittest, fight or flight perspective. Our first symbols emphasize "fortakeness." They are the mental equivalents of nature's repertoire of physical behavior. Symbolic dominance and aggression are an alternative to physical dominance and aggression. Physical might is replaced by economic, political, and/ or religious symbols of power – money, expensive "toys," titles, "beauty," approval, patriotism, and a variety of symbolic rewards limited only by our imagination. Hatred, resentment, jealousy, greed, and the like become the symbolic replacements for fighting.

Would you now envision that in just the manner we organize our symbols to create harmful aggression to dominate and control others, this same resource is available to us to create love, cooperation, sharing, philanthropy, happiness, peace of mind, and yes, even peace in the world. **These positive qualities of our manner of thinking are quite difficult to create when our thinking is occupied with the first manner of harmful aggression we acquire as part of our nature. Forgiveness is a basic mental strength that allows us to move on to those mental "magical" uses of symbols that express constructive use of our aggressive energy.** For this reason, forgiveness is one of our most powerful assets.

Forgiveness, like love, is quite rare in our world compared to our preoccupation with the *fortakeness* expressed in the various forms of harmful aggression mentioned above. I believe we may each acquire skill in directing our thinking to love and forgive. The secret is to practice *self*-endorsement. We will continue to have great difficulty giving to others what we lack in ourselves. This is why the Guide emphasizes practical strens on *self*-endorsement. I believe we are fully capable of manufacturing love as we manufacture hate. However, directing our mental energy to constructive aggression is a skill that must be cultivated, unlike the destructive bent that is pre-wired into our thinking by our trial-and-error genetic history. I hope this theory stren will motivate you to attend to the skills of love and forgiveness. I, and you, and our world benefit by every individual who converts their mental manufacturing plant to produce love more so than the harmful aggression.

Before leaving this consideration of forgiveness, I want to address a common misconception. Forgiveness is not meant to free others or ourselves from responsibility; it does not excuse harmful action. In addition to freeing our *self* from energy draining preoccupation such as resentment, forgiveness redirects our innate responses that call for punishment and destructive aggression to instead provide education, rehabilitation, problem-solving, and appropriate limit-setting. It allows us to address the issue in a manner that has the most productive outcome for all parties. The distinction between punishment and limit-setting is subtle but significant.[5]

----

[5] See the stren *Good Aggression*, Chapter 3 available in the full course on the Internet at *www.anwot.org*.

7. MY "REACT BUTTON" FANTASY

This stren deals with taking greater control of your*self*.

As a result of my observations of people, I have come to imagine that all of us have, coming from our mid-sections, a large button sticking out far in front. I call this button a "React Button" because someone or some situation may come along, trigger the button, and SNAP! We regularly automatically react in a characteristic way to the outside event. I see some of us as being so sensitive and reactive that we have additional React Buttons on our backs, sides, even "all over." Perhaps you know such super-reactive persons.

The situation goes like this: There is an unpleasant event or act by an "other." Frustration understandably occurs, and the person may not only overreact at the time but also allows the event to get them stuck in *self*-defeating emotions ... resentment, irritability, self-pity, lethargy, withdrawal, physical symptoms, and so on. The person's button is pushed and the person dwells in the "injustice" in such a way that no good comes of it.

Most of us allow our React Buttons to be exposed to a number of people and circumstances. Take a few moments to think of a few situations in which you permit your button to be pushed. Think about the important people in your life -- family, friends, anyone you've worked with or for. Can you visualize the size and number of <u>their</u> React Buttons? Kids react buttons are often the most obvious – "No, I won't buy you that toy." They really <u>are</u> dependent!

In order to take charge of our responses to life's frustration, we need to develop the adult skill of "pulling in, hand-over-hand," our React Button(s) and getting our OWN hand on it. Thus, when an event occurs that would have formerly, automatically triggered the button, instead of reacting, we act.[6] Responding with action involves thinking before following the old pattern or <u>reacting</u>.   It means delaying long enough to ask our *self*, "What is the long-term consequence I would choose to occur?" or, "What steps on my part are most likely to get me where I wish to go?" This involves *self*-control, rather than following

---

[6] One person remarked, "Not reacting is being inhuman." Teaching our self to recognize and restrain our first level reaction is not to be confused with the state of being nonresponsive, Pollyannaish, or insensitive. We generally arrive at our wisest response pattern when reflection guides us to self-directed ACTION (the alternative to automatic REACTION). This distinction was brought out in a discussion with a nurse during a staff conference. She said, "I like to be sensitive and in touch with my feelings, to let go of my emotions, to laugh, cry, to shout. I like being spontaneous. I don't want to be nonreactive."
"Then do you allow yourself to respond emotionally all the time?" I asked.
"Oh, no. I choose to let go when I think the situation is appropriate, with some of the staff in certain situations." Most of us recognize that we increase our coping capability when we possess the skill to CHOOSE how and when to express our feelings.
The key to self-control is being consciously aware of our feelings and CHOOSING how and when to express them appropriately. In some situations we express our feelings spontaneously; at other times we appropriately delay and hold on. The skill here is in choosing how we "explode" or "let go" in automatic response to the "other." In accepting responsibility for our self, we learn to keep our hand on our React Button; we don't turn it over to the "other." Are you mostly a "holder-on-er," a "let-go-er," or do you choose your response wisely?

some habitual computer-type program. We may think about and then even choose the same action response as if we had simply reacted without thinking; this would, however, be a conscious, deliberate, likely wiser, choice-among-alternatives rather than a passive turning-over the control of our feelings to another.

Please understand that our reactions are automatic *first level responses* that are usually helpful in emergency situations, such as withdrawing our hand from a hot surface or striking our arm when we feel the mosquito bite. They are related to our innate "fight or flight" behavior to protect our life and well-being. However, in today's relatively civilized world, we rarely face emergency situations. Fighting or running or their symbolic counterparts of verbally attacking others (or our *self*) are generally not productive. Indeed, blaming, resentment, self-putdowns, prolonged worry and anxiety are commonly the life's discomforts <u>we</u> inflict on our *self*. Expect the first level automatic reaction, label it, and then contemplate appropriate action. At issue is avoiding getting stuck in reaction.

Example: John worked diligently and effectively helping his employer's business grow. He was on track to become vice-president - so he thought.   How frustrated when he was told the owner was bringing in his green and undeserving nephew to be vice president. Yes, John experienced the hurt of this major setback. But he didn't let himself get stuck in any of the multiple negative reactions that would have added to his upset and make himself his own enemy. Rather he thought through his alternatives - speak with the owner and negotiate some degree of justice, i.e., his best deal, decide to make the best of the situation and consider making a new opportunity in another job, and enthusiastically carry on the many other aspects of his life.

We are innately prone to react when someone does what we don' like or something happens that is unpleasant. Consider this: every time we allow our React Button to be pushed, we are turning our *self* over to someone or something and allowing the "other" to determine how we feel or what we do. We are saying, in effect, "Here, you hold my button. You take control of me!"   It's difficult enough that we do suffer the consequences of the negative event; do we benefit by continuing our day with preoccupation, *self*-pity, resentment, and the like? This is like going to the market, buying something, paying for it, and then ... going back and paying for it again and again! Is this what we really desire? Yet, my observation is that we do this frequently without even thinking about it.

Freedom, which we highly prize and strive for is the opportunity to choose among alternatives. **To the degree your React Button is sticking out, you will be the slave to whomever or whatever pushes it. Think about that!**

I have been pleased to observe many individuals who, with simple awareness of this fantasy and a bit of practical application, dramatically increase their self-control. They gradually learn to ACT instead of REACT and delightedly find that their fate is no longer so dependent on other people or on life events over which they have no control.

Read this "React Button" fantasy and it won't help you. But if you read it regularly in an attempt to understand it, and then practice applying it day-by-day, it'll do wonders!

You have just received a PEARL! Know it! Use it! You'll enjoy it!

[This stren complements the *Blaming Mental Response Pattern (MRP)*, the most common of the eight choices available to our will in transforming information into action. You will receive this stren in section 5 beginning on page 49]

SECTION THREE ▮

8. A VOCABULARY STREN: EITHER...OR; BOTH...AND

This stren is likely the most powerful to develop a newer way of thinking (ANWOT). It is the basis of mature thinking and the elimination of prejudice (pre-judgment).

*A great many people think they are thinking when
they are merely rearranging their prejudices. William James*

The instructions are clear. The application is easy. The results are profound. **Simply attempt to substitute "both...and" for "either...or" each and every time it makes sense to do so.**

Throughout our early years, when we are physically immature and mentally undeveloped, we learn to think in terms of "either...or." We divide the world into me or not me, us or them, friend or foe, right or wrong, good or bad, O.K. or not O.K., yes or no (we mostly say "yes," our parents say "no!"), can or can't, for me or against me, safe or dangerous, and so on. Processing information into two categories is called "dichotomous thinking." After thousands of repetitions, dichotomous thinking becomes wired into our native language and becomes the effortless habitual manner we process information to action. It is self-evident that this early manner of categorizing data into two categories distorts our perception of the world. Labels like *bad, wrong, ugly,* turn-on prejudice, intolerance, hatred, and related blaming behaviors. Do you see how our early manner of thinking is a common source of conflict? We regularly observe instances of dichotomous thinking persisting in adults, law[7], aesthetics, religion, and communication between nations. Limiting our alternatives to two categories restricts our creative thinking just as I would be limited in writing this stren if my computer was equipped with a *spreadsheet* software program and had no *word* processing program or a very primitive one.

We may produce a cup of coffee by heating four distinct ingredients: ground coffee beans, water, milk, and sugar. The product is no longer the distinct ingredients but a mixture of $a + b + c + d$. The interaction of our genes, nurturers, and *self*; of instinct, habit, and will, and their means of expression, i.e. their "operating systems" (O.S.s), is likewise a mixture with characteristics distinctive from the original ingredients. With the cup of coffee, we may start with only water and coffee, and choose to add a fraction of milk or make the drink mostly milk; we can add a little sugar, a cup of sugar, or no sugar. The

---

[7] Our criminal justice system has traditionally been based on "Innocent or guilty?" Where are the shades of gray?

combinations are infinite. Similarly, can you imagine that biologic creatures first function according to the rules of nature? To nature's rules, nurturers may add a little or quite a bit. And to the mixture of nature and nurture, we may add a little or quite a lot of our *self*. In each situation, there is a continuum of variation. The product of mixing the rules of our genes, our nurturers, and our *self* also has infinite combinations. We are prone to distort reality when we think in terms of <u>either</u> *a* <u>or</u> *b* <u>or</u> *c*. We are usually more accurate when we think in terms of "both...and": *a* <u>and</u> *b* <u>and</u> *c*. While the majority of earth's creatures are mostly nature-driven, humans receive a huge dose of programming from nurturers, and in our later stage of development we add *self*-direction.

Such often-asked questions as, "What's more important, nature <u>or</u> nurture?" and "Which came first, the chicken <u>or</u> the egg?" distorts our understanding. This is an appropriate question from an immature mind that yet thinks in "either...or" terms. We can picture change occurring in a continuous spiral, first something like the chicken, then something like the egg, progressing to what we now recognize as the chicken and the egg. We recognize that the early instances of phenomena are usually primitive and gradually evolve to become what we recognize now in its advanced stage. "Simple" usually increases in complexity and/or efficiency over time. Knowledge, reason, and wisdom are acquired only after considerable physical and mental maturity. Updating our thinking by emphasizing *both... and* allows us to get beyond our primitive *either...or* first manner of processing information.

We have no difficulty choosing between a garbage sandwich and a sandwich containing a favorite food. In actuality, the complex world we live in seldom presents such simple choices. We view the menu of a restaurant; choice-making requires weighing the positives and negatives of each alternative. We can be happy with most of the alternatives. The choice of spending <u>or</u> saving our money has pluses and minuses on each side. Wisdom may suggest we do both, save some <u>and</u> spend some. Similarly, most issues, such as ethics and aesthetics, are not *right* or *wrong*. They also usually present us with a combination of positives and negatives. Is a concerned mother who steals milk so her child can survive a sinner <u>or</u> a saint? Neither? Right <u>or</u> wrong? Good <u>or</u> bad? Are our enemies "all" wrong, evil, while we are "all" right and just in our cause? Does our manner of thinking allow us to recognize that the "other" often has similar needs, wants, and passion for love, justice, and peace as we do? We may wisely ask how much does our manner of thinking contribute to our <u>making</u> the other our enemy? To what degree would we be wise to emphasize *making our choices right* more so than *making the right choice*?

Dichotomous thinking is black or white. ANWOT thinking is in Technicolor! Here is an example:

> *There is so much bad in the best of us,*
> *And so much good in the worst of us,*
> *That it ill behooves any of us,*
> *To put down the rest of us.*

We act wisely when we update our thinking with Technicolor!

To the degree we limit our thinking to *either...or*, we predictably distort our commonly-shared reality to suit our personal bias. There are wiser more accurate alternatives. Nevertheless, our innate dichotomous thinking, reinforced by repetition, remains the preferred path information is processed. Considerable practice is required to substitute the more productive manner of thinking.

We can understand and forgive our nurturers. They teach us to think in *either...or* terms when we are mentally immature and physically undeveloped, when we are unable to determine when to cross the street, touch the stove, and to not wipe our nose on the curtain. Most mean well and do their reasonable best with what their pupils can manage. When we attain maturity, we often remain imperceptibly stuck in our early manner of thinking. The newer manner of thinking is attained by those fortunate to have wise role models, and/or who just "get it" through common sense and experience. For most, dichotomous thinking and/or its remnants are a major source of prejudice, intolerance, hatred, and destructive acts of aggression.

The problem remains huge because our culture has yet to provide the simple educational resources that teach us how to upgrade our manner of thinking. Do you realize that in every reasonable size city, one can open a phone book and/or turn on the TV and find instruction in physical exercise, computers, real estate, poker, playing a musical instrument and very esoteric subjects? Yet where does one turn to learn the most basic skills of constructive thinking? As need is recognized, solutions usually follow. I envision that we will spawn various forms of education in ANWOT in the near future.

The cure for dichotomous thinking is readily acquired by anyone willing to engage in a simple mental exercise. It requires substituting an *analog*[8] word or trigger-switch[9] such as *both...and* for the prevalent dichotomous *either...or* words. This easy step, regularly practiced, will promote our well-being. Practiced by many, it will also improve our community's well-being.

Both...and and *either...or* are trigger-switches. They each trigger the pathway through which thinking leads to action. *Both...and* channels thinking to follow the preferred updated pathway of *self*-mastery. *Either...or* directs energy along the wiring pre-established by our genes and nurturers. Keep in mind that the prejudices, the "pre-judgments" of nature are designed to emphasize the immediate short-term solution, to satisfy "me" often at the expense of "not me." Nature's perspective is amoral.

---

[8] The following example helps me understand how *analog* differs from dichotomous. The old fashioned watches were analog. Their hands moved continuously around the clock. The newer digital watches are dichotomous. The hand jumps to be on 1 or 2 or 3 and so on. The digital movement is *either...or* more so than the analog watch which misses nothing between. The analog movement continuously adds to what was; it is this and that, not this or that.

[9] A trigger-switch is a word(s) that, like a light switch, turns-*on* or *off* the manner energy is directed to an action outcome. By substituting appropriate trigger words for those imbedded in our native language we may redirect our thinking to preferred outcomes. The limited number of *self*-mastery trigger words identified in this Guide updates our thinking to have a huge influence in attaining thought control.

Our nurturers' prejudices, their pre-judgments, are likewise dictatorial. The dichotomous perspective our nurturers inscribe in us through our immature years may convey immense wisdom, absolute compliance, and/or anything in between, depending on how fate has selected *their* nurturers. Though predictably well-meaning, we can be certain their best efforts apply to the circumstances of their own nurturing and require updating, especially with the rapidly accelerating changes we now initiate through science. When we jump immediately to the *either...or* manner of processing information before considering *both...and*, before using our reflective thinking skills, we yet submit our creativity to the whims of fate and circumstance. Blind obedience is unacceptable to a freed mind.

Earth's creatures have passively evolved adhering to the rules provided by instinct and habit. Nature provides us a magnificent brain. Our nurturers equip it with sophisticated language. In the course of attaining maturity, we combine these two marvelous resources to become proficient in reflective thinking, the ability to think about our thinking, to be conscious of our consciousness. While reflective thinking is nature's and our nurturers' gift of opportunity, the mental freedom to direct our will power requires our own doing. We bear the responsibility to emancipate our will from what fate and circumstance have made of us. We also make the choice of what degree of wisdom to add, even to determine <u>what</u> is "wise."

As our use of language, originality, and creativity has grown, and with it our growth of power and collection of wisdom, we can recognize the benefit of updating the means we process information, of adding ANWOT. We are rapidly increasing our freedom to modify the programs of nature and nurture, and to initiate new programs within our mental operating system. Skillful reflective thinking enables our *self* to join and mitigate the persuasive power of nature and nurture to direct our life's experience.

As our *self* emerges it may add reason and wisdom to instinct and habit. The wise use of reason requires newer means of processing information to action, ANWOT. If we choose to develop a newer way of thinking, we are required to challenge our established patterns. Nature, through genes, first programs our thinking. Our nurturers challenge and significantly modify the patterns of instinct we inherit. The challenge to our *self* is to add reason, self-initiation, originality, creativity, and constructive leadership to our resource for reflective thinking. Let's update the means for processing information-to-action acquired from our first masters and make them appropriate for modernity.

Now to avoid confusion, let us clarify that *either...or* may indeed be very appropriate <u>after</u> we wisely consider the *both...and*, pluses <u>and</u> minuses, positives <u>and</u> negatives of each of our alternatives. By doing so, we are far more likely to problem-solve with a better understanding of reality, make wiser choices, and assume short <u>and</u> long-term responsibility for our choice-making.

Self-management is a powerful tool for constructive <u>and</u> destructive action. It surely will be disastrous in a mind stuck in dichotomous thinking. The importance of taking action to educate ourselves in the skill of wise thinking is self-evident. **You will take an important simple step by substituting** *both ... and* **thinking for** *either ... or* **thinking whenever it is reasonable.**

SUMMARY: Our first manner of thinking divides the world into two categories. Generally whatever is *me* is good, right, and praiseworthy. Whatever is *not me* should be for my benefit or it is bad, wrong, and deserving of harm. Genes prepare us to instinctively fight or run to preserve our *self*. Our nurturers instill in our mind what is good, right, needed to win and dominate; and with it, we recognize their opposites … what is bad, wrong, the losers who are unworthy. Our current establishment is deficient in educating its citizens how to update our thinking for modernity. Until ANWOT is routinely taught, we can expect continuation of harmful prejudice, hatred, intolerance, and waste of our valuable energy on destructive aggression. As we recognize our manner of thinking is the main source of our problems, we will initiate the rapid growth of learning opportunities in the newer way of thinking, in ANWOT.

----

9. Cash in Your Anger

This vocabulary stren explains how to trade-in the anger (that gets you what you don't want) for energy to buy what really works. A few basic mental skills will redirect aggressive energy from <u>de</u>structive to <u>con</u>structive outcomes.

Every person in every culture throughout the world experiences anger. We've all seen examples of very explosive anger. Many persons are "loaded" but hardly outwardly express their anger. Resentment, guilting one's self, muscle tension (viz. backaches and headaches, teeth grinding), elevated blood pressure, and/or becoming an alcoholic or workaholic are among the many ways anger gets directed. How do you express your anger? Wouldn't you like to trade in your anger for energy that really works <u>for</u> you? It's easy if you just apply what you already have. Wow! Anger is our most important source of wealth, if we only spend it wisely. **Here are the simple mental changes that update our thinking to thrive in our contemporary society.**

   a. **Substitute the word** *energy* **each time you experience what you now call** *anger*.
   b. **Immediately follow your label** *energy* **with the magical problem-solving mental**
      response: *Given this situation* (which indeed may be quite unfair and unpleasant), *what is most likely to get me what I want for now <u>and</u> the future, for me <u>and</u> you* (or *for us <u>and</u> them; that may also benefit the 'other')?* This sentence directs our thinking to see our *self* as a member of the larger system of which we are a part and to consider the future as well as immediate consequences of action. Most all wise action is preceded by mental rehearsal and problem-solving.
   c. **Substitute the word** *urgency* **when you experience** *emergency* **and assign** *high,* *medium,* **or** *low priority*.

That's it! Try it … it works. Here's why:

Nature, through our genes and our chemical makeup, viz. DNA, provides us and every living creature with energy. Energy is the stuff we use to get what we need. Our first need is survival; otherwise we wouldn't be here. Nature also programs us with survival behaviors. Fight and/or flight are among our most powerfully built-in survival behaviors. Over billions of years of evolution, nature's way has emphasized fighting and/ or running to get food, to mate and protect our young, and to keep us from becoming food.

In our relatively civilized society, fighting and/or running rarely get us what we want. More often, some form of hurt or punishment is the outcome. I know of and have personally spoken with many persons who have long, even lifetime jail terms for a single impulsive act of rage, often totally out of context with their usual behavior. You have surely observed the negative consequences of anger in others. Can you think of acts of anger that you wish <u>you</u> could take back? Anger is a trigger-switch[10] whose most common pathway leads to nature's pre-wired manner of processing energy to harmful aggression. Thus anger commonly triggers the primitive *mental* response pattern (MRP) I call *Blaming*. *Blaming-out* and/or *Blaming-in* both usually result in an emergency response to strike out, to engage in <u>de</u>structive physical and/or mental aggression. What words might pop into your mind when a driver cuts you off, someone outright lies to you, or upon some injustice you currently face or have experienced? When you make a really big mistake? Though "standard" in primitive creatures, the pattern of *need/want → arousal (frustration) → aggression → striking-out* is rarely productive in our relatively civilized society. Anger is commonly followed by aggressive acts that get us what we <u>don't</u> want. However, aggression need not be harmful! Aggressive energy may be redirected to "do good" more so than do harm.

Our nurturers usually teach us to redirect our bent for physical aggression to symbolic aggression. We learn such mental means as to blame (often our *self*), resent, win by "beating" others in competition, dominate and lord over others with wealth, status, titles, "rightness," and asserting that God and/or whatever the prevailing power must be is on our side. We learn to name our energy "anger". Anger ("I am angry!") is a trigger word that sets-off our most primitive physical and/or mental means of reaction. It commonly and effortlessly sets-off the **blaming <u>M</u>ental <u>R</u>esponse <u>P</u>attern (MRP):** *Someone or something did wrong; therefore they deserve harm,* **and/or** *I did wrong and therefore I deserve harm.* Anger is thus expressed as harmful aggression. Can you see that destructive physical and mental aggression is routinely wired into our native language and the way we think, i.e. how we process information to action? Herein is the major source of prejudice, hatred, and the direction of our creative energy to destructive aggression, including war. So it is unless and/or until we teach ourselves a better way.

We each have the opportunity to update our manner of processing information to consistently attain constructive outcomes. **Simply substitute the trigger-word** *energy* **for the trigger-word** *anger.* **Immediately and habitually follow** *energy* **with the magical** *problem-solving MRP* **instead of the** *blaming MRP.* The problem-solving sentence is not magic but it works so well it will seem magical. And once made habitual through repetition, the newer problem-solving response will appear automatically with little conscious effort. It will replace the blaming response that becomes habitual within the native language we acquire over 16 or so years of physical and mental immaturity.

---

[10] A trigger-switch, like a light switch, provides direction for a specific manner of processing energy. The few preferred trigger or word-switches identified in this <u>Guide</u> update our thinking to have a huge influence in attaining thought control and *self*-mastery.

Emergencies: Nature has programmed our body to respond to most frustration and threat as an emergency. Our bodies are genetically designed for immediate reflex action. For most creatures, the automatic response of fight or flight is life-saving. One mishap can be fatal. Thus, our physical emergency response is powerful and ever present. When we perceive threat, frustration, and/or need, raw energy for action is produced. Our body responds with automatic biologic changes. Adrenalin, sugar and "action" substances are released. Heart rate and blood pressure increase. Blood is diverted to muscles and our brain and away from routine maintenance issues such as digestion and sexual interest. Irrespective of race, religion, gender, or color, we each inherit this gift from nature.

Since frustration is a normal part of our life's experience and we are mentally prone to perceive stresses as threats, we can count on frequent activation of our emergency response. Blaming, resentment, and hatred sustain our short-term **red alert** tension state as an ongoing unhealthy **pink alert** state. Even though our **red alert** is frequently triggered, virtually every experience is a false alarm! Emergency reactions to nonemergency situations seldom get us what we want. And maintaining a state of **pink alert** may contribute to elevated blood pressure, muscle contraction pain, impaired sleep, digestive and sexual dysfunction, and/or a host of other physiologic maladies. We best learn to update management of our inherent fight response to effectively deal with the unprecedented types of challenges we confront in our contemporary society.

Most unhappiness and stress is related to our manner of thinking. Too often <u>we</u> are our own worst enemy. This is very good news because it means we are in the best position to prevent what we bring on our *self*. Our innate and first acquired response system, once effective, is likely to bring harm more so than relief. I have heard many wise people say: "Don't sweat the small issues … and almost <u>all</u> issues are small!" **By substituting** *urgent* **for** *emergency* **and assigning the issue** *high, medium,* **or** *low priority,* **we more efficiently and productively manage our life's experiences.** *Urgent* **conveys to us that the issue may be important but need not require immediate action.** Consider that the "emergency" issues we face in today's world, such as the environment, weapons of mass destruction, poverty, religious conflict, and so on require creative problem-solving, negotiation, patience, and resources unlike the automatic fight and/or flight response applicable in primitive societies. Our contemporary stresses are best resolved with planning, knowledge, manipulation of ideas, and mentally rehearsing alternative actions before initiating which of the alternatives we deem wisest.

The substitute trigger-words *energy* for *anger*, and *urgent* for *emergency*, will be appropriate in virtually every instance. Misdirected anger can cause irreparable harm in a very short time. *Prevention* surely beats *cure!* **A simple word change often results in a dramatic change in perspective, meaning, interpretation, and action outcome.** Words wired to habitual pathways that stimulate rational problem-solving stimulate behaviors that support a civilized, peace-loving society. Let's harness the energy we commonly waste on destructive and/or nonproductive aggression to attain our desired goals. Practice prevention by telling yourself repeatedly, "Rarely are there emergencies!" until it pops up easily when your **red-alert** button is pushed. Add, "I am wise to think about this to consider alternatives and then decide what action to take."

Teaching our *self* to routinely recognize our anger and direct its energy using the problem-solving mental response rewards us with constructive outcomes we can enjoy throughout our lifetime. With practice, substituting the trigger-word *energy* for *anger*, applying the problem-solving sentence, and assigning priority to dealing with your issues will become a coordinated effortless action. Give yourself regular bonuses! – Endorse yourself with enthusiasm each time you redirect your anger to problem-solving. Do cash in your anger for the much more valuable energy and enjoy your newfound wealth! The strens *The Mental Response Control Panel*, and *MRCP Step 2*, explains the other mental choices available to us. The strens on blaming will explain how to avoid the most common thinking that gets us into trouble.

Global change: As you grow skill in managing your aggressive energy, you will become a missionary of constructive aggression, a soldier in the army fighting the pervasive destructive aggression we view daily. Progress in spreading the newer way of thinking is made one + one + one; *each one, teach one.*

Summary: Here is the simple recipe to convert destructive aggression to the energy we require to feel good and "do good."

What to do: Substitute a "label" for your present emergency response that is less associated with *harm* than anger. *Energy* is such a word; it is more suggestive of *creativity* than *harm*. When possible, replace habitually established words that trigger harmful action such as **anger, resentment, and/or anxiety[11] with *energy*!** Changing the label we assign to our high arousal experience can make a dramatic difference in our perspective. *Anger* is commonly pre-wired to set off destructive aggression. *Energy* (unlike *anger, resentment,* or *anxiety*) is neutral. It conveys greater freedom of choice in directing action. It directs our thinking to process information through a newer creative mental pathway that leads to a beneficial outcome. **This easy *energy* substitution can then be made a signal to automatically call forth the problem-solving sentence.** Reflective thinking is most likely to result in wise resolution of an urgent issue, more so than the harmful physical and/or mental aggression that commonly leads to escalation. *Self-mastery* favors the problem-solving response, i.e. mental rehearsal of alternatives to consider long-term as well as short-term outcomes ... and wisdom to challenge impulsive blaming. Initial attempts to break the old "anger" habit pattern will be challenging. However, after clumsy efforts, and with practice, the newer <u>constructive</u> direction of energy will become automatic and effortless.

**Periodically remind your*self*: *real emergencies are rare.* With repetition, we can establish the habit of thinking and using the problem-solving mental response pattern (MRP) <u>prior</u> to impulsive action. In our contemporary society, rage and reactive behavior most commonly reflect turning over control of our emotions to some "other," just what we don't want. Our innate proneness to deal with challenges as an emergency rarely serves its original purpose. We are wise to modify it. Mental rehearsal applying the problem-<u>solving sentence</u> constructively directs our energy to both short and long-term solutions.

---

[11] If we mentally strip away the urge to strike out and sustain this alerting response with "what if's," the arousal of energy experience is more likely to be labeled anxiety instead of anger. "What if" thinking is a major source of incapacitating phobias and anxiety attacks.

SECTION FOUR ▌

10. <u>YOUR LOVE-MAKING FACTORY – BECOMING A BETTER LOVER</u>

This stren provides a view of love and is an introduction to the skill of becoming **your own best friend.** It can improve your lovemaking (LM) - to yourself, and to others.

Likely you know one or more persons who have a great capacity to express love; and likely you can think of some others who have a great capacity to be hateful. So much of our energy that goes into producing love or hate can be under our direct control - we can have immense say in the degree we love and hate and in what form we choose to express our self. The testimonial of others, personal experience and observation, verify the importance of love to a fulfilling life. This stren offers directions in growing your love-making ability. We lack disciplined teaching programs to develop LM skills (do you agree?). This is an attempt to fill this void. This theory stren provides an understanding of *making* love; the practical strens provide the "how to" steps.

On love:

Many persons I have asked to express what love is, respond saying they don't know how to describe it but they "know what it is." The disciplined teaching and learning of a skill (here the skill of making love) requires identification; "Learning starts with labeling." Let's begin by attempting to identify the skill of creating "love."

I distinguish 3 types. Erotic love originates in our genes to insure reproduction. The "filial" love we have as a parent is a second type. While parental caring is also biologically motivated (it may be turned "on" or "off" in most life by a hormone), in creatures having a long period of dependence, such as ourselves, the love of a parent for a child is mostly learned from our nurturers. The third type of mature love is that which we our *self* make, independent of what our nature or nurture provides. Of these three sources of love – nature, nurture, and our *self*, this stren focuses on the "mature love" we our *self* create. [A son urged me to call this "love-creation" instead of "love-making" to distinguish it from our common association of love-making as a sexual act. If you prefer, simply substitute "LC" when I refer to "LM."]

Love is energy and attention directed for the benefit of someone (including yourself!) and/or something beyond one's self. Love is not of a limited quantity; we can make a little, a lot, or virtually none. An eight-child parent is not restricted to give 1/8th the love to each child that a one-child parent can offer. Indeed, each of the eight children in a family may receive more love than the only child in a family. Likewise, you may love (and/or hate) an "other," many "others," and you may love your*self*. Giving love to one friend doesn't mean you need love another less.

Love is a willing gift, i.e. you have great freedom to generate love and decide where and how you direct it. Your loving may be short or long-lived. Your loving may continue, cease, increase, or decrease, in the same manner a factory may increase, decrease, or cease production, and the factory (as you yourself) may even change what it is producing. Indeed, this stren proposes that you review the products coming from your energy factory and increase your loving capacity.

What thoughts do you hold about love? How do your views agree? Differ? Most religions and ethical programs teach that you love your neighbor as yourself. What does this mean to you?

Qualities of a lover*:

Pure love requires the maturity to enjoy giving without strings, i.e., there is satisfaction in the act of giving even when the act of loving is not returned. The gift of love is a complete act in itself. The lover has learned to love him/her self and is skillfully self-endorsing. It is difficult to give with an empty cup. When you first fill your cup and it overflows, you then have the greatest capacity to give. [The person who gives with an unfilled cup often resents the receiver when the response is less than expected.] The love-maker skillfully uses energy to enrich others, and the world we share...and experiences joy in so doing. He/she has become aware of his/her natural tendency to blame, recognizes and redirects this energy in a positive direction.

The lover may have very limited or immense capacity. Most religions and cultures have examples of infinite lovers, for example, Jesus. While one may strive to be an infinite lover, reality suggests that doing our "reasonable best" is a practical obtainable goal. To me, this means allocating an appropriate amount of our energy to continued growth of our LM capacity and being sufficiently humble to accept our human limitations and fallibility.

*This stren primarily focuses on the creation of love. The capacities to express love and to receive love are important qualities mentioned here but more directly addressed elsewhere.

1. In my observation, many persons create and feel their love but have great difficulty expressing it. It is as though we have a rationed quantity of love and we'd better store it for when we really need it. The words "I love you" are rarely expressed. Quite obtuse ways are devised to express love in a manner that would not hurt if the loved one doesn't "properly" receive our love. In a recent popular sitcom, Raymond is asked by his wife why he never says "I love you." Though he quite obviously does, he chokes on the word and finally says, "I show you with my eyes."

2. While the mature lover derives joy in his/her act of giving love and isn't giving merely to get, the capacity to receive love is also a most worthy quality of LM. Recognize that the loved person's acceptance and acknowledgment of the love offered by another is itself an act of loving; it does enrich the satisfaction of even the most experienced lover ... AND is immeasurably encouraging to the novice lover in his/her tender often clumsy attempts to grow their LM factory. To maintain unconditional loving is a very advanced skill few attain; thus, the gracious acceptance of the givers gift is your gift. [I have observed many persons who become quite good lovers but have little capacity to graciously accept love.]

Do you agree with this description? What would you add? Subtract? How do you assess your own LM skills?

Your love-making factory, and steps to strengthen it:
Picture within your*self* the energy factory that carries out your life's activities. Making love is among the many skillfully created products of your factory. [What other products can you identify: viz. hate? jealousy[12]? worry? greed? knowledge? ideas? music? material products?] Your factory production is determined by a Board of Directors; it consists of your genes (what you need), your nurturers (what you are expected to want), and your*self* (what is wise). There is a chief executive officer (CEO) of your Board of Directors who has the last word. And though you may become CEO of your energy factory's production, you would be unwise to assume this powerful position without appropriate skill. Consider your lack of such skills when you came into this world and the multiple years nature and/or your nurturers served as CEO to make you what you are. [Who have been and still are on your current Board of Directors?[13]] Much of the early teachings we receive not only don't contribute to becoming CEO of our factory, they are persuasive in immobilizing such aspirations. Realize that you can learn to wisely direct what and how much your factory produces. This *taking charge* process has been referred to elsewhere as "becoming your own person." We learn from those who have developed such skills, have clarified the resources needed, and may also be worthy role models (that's what strens are about). You are on you way to being CEO when you become aware of the factory within you and grow your response ability to make a difference.

You pick which TV station you watch, you may choose to develop a job skill, study a language, or learn to play a musical instrument, AND you have the resources to grow your love-making factory. Now let's focus on the LM portion of your energy factory and consider the resources needed to "turn on" your production.

LM is a skill that you may choose to study, learn, and develop. You have a good start if you have been lucky enough to have experienced loving role models. Disciplined preparation in "loving" has long been neglected; most persons could far better explain how to play bingo than how to create love. We receive far more instruction in reading, job training, and so much else. To grow your LM, you will likely need to make room in your factory and re-direct some of your attention and energy, i.e., a willingness to challenge and let go of old established habits that don't get you what you want, and frequently get you what you don't want.

---

[12] Jealousy may be just behind prejudice as a major source of destructive aggression.

[13] Chapter 4, B. and C. in the full course will help you identify the important members of your Board.

Action begins with the faith that "Yes, I can." The ingredients to growing your LM factory are all available to you. You have or can surely acquire the five needed ingredients -- faith in your capacity to make a difference, work (practice), direction, patience, and risk-taking[14] (willingness to let go of some old patterns to focus on creating love, factory space if you will). Superior intelligence, wealth, and even good health are not required. Absolutely zero (0) magic is needed though new skills may seem to work magically. Like any skill, growing your LM factory is acquired step-by-step, in bits and pieces. Some bits are best acquired before you can master the more advanced pieces that contribute to your LM production.

The main intent of this stren is that you become aware of your LM factory and your capacity to invest your energy in its development. Thereby, you can proceed to acquire the additional "strengths" or multiple skills that grow your LM factory. Each skill is teachable and learnable. You can surely develop these skills. In my efforts at growing my own LM factory, I have identified many component skills that I have described in additional strens that are available to you. These components of growing your LM factory are briefly elaborated in the Addendum accompanying this stren. These "bits and pieces" useful for growing your LM factory emphasize self-endorsement - becoming your own best friend (a very basic skill worthy of your earliest attention!), learning from mistakes, acquiring the vocabulary of mature thinking, recognizing and dealing with blaming (resentments, jealousy, destructive aggression), using the near magical problem solving sentence, strengthening faith – the "yes I can" skill, the skill of forgiving, the "reasonable best" measure of your self-worth (avoiding perfectionism), patience, dealing with anxiety, clarifying your values, and ultimately your skill to create new strens that are most meaningful to you and that may also make a difference as you share them with others. The strens here identified are picked from a larger collection because they most directly contribute to developing your LM factory. Though often not specific to LM; they will contribute in other ways to your skill in the management of your life, to feeling good and doing good.

Love and sex (here mentioned because they are often confused):
Love and sex have distinct qualities. They can be experienced together or separately. Together, they can be glorious and mutually enhancing. Though our language commonly associates them, they need not go together ... (like bacon and eggs; health, wealth and happiness; parenthood, responsibility and commitment; religion, faith and peace of mind).

Sexual gratification is primarily a *response* from direct stimulation of nerve endings, which is conveyed to a relatively primitive area of the brain and is thereafter experienced consciously (in our newer brain). Interest characteristically is heightened at puberty with hormonal and physical changes, is sustained as a powerful instinctual drive, and often declines with the hormonal and physical changes of aging. It is of considerable interest that the sexual pleasure area of our more primitive "automatic" brain is closely intertwined with the area for aggression. This makes sense because a species would not exist without a compelling drive to aggressively seek pleasure and procreate.[15] Our genitals and skin

---

[14] These five ingredients and their ready availability are explained in other strens.

[15] Consider how our behavior might change if babies were born instantly and orgasm came nine months later.

contain receptors that *receive* information whereas love is willfully *transmitted*. Sexual fulfillment may be very non-discriminating towards whom or what is providing the stimulation. Love, while having powerful emotional ties, is more strongly influenced by the last to develop cortical "thinking" portion of the brain, what I call our *freedom organ*. And while loving actions may be acquired from role models, LM is a more conscious "willing" *act* growing with mental and emotional maturity, and the development of our skill in reflective thinking. Infatuation may be a mental and emotional by-product of sexual or other emotions, but does not have the same voluntary giving quality as love.

Do we "fall in love" or *crawl into love*? The distinction is important! Here is my explanation. "Falling" is governed by gravity, a force outside of our jurisdiction. "Crawling" is powered by our own will, an act we choose. Nature has deemed procreation basic to survival of a species. It so powerfully "machines" its subjects to engage in reproductive activity that copulation is ritualistically pursued even when life itself is at risk. This is especially clear in the animal kingdom. Genes overlap aggression and pleasure centers in the primitive portion of all brains, add features designed to attract a mate, and chemicals to assure newborns will be nurtured to a state of self-survival. Nature demands that we "fall into sex." We also call this "infatuation" and/or mistakenly "love." Unconditional concern for the "other" is often not part of nature's plan.

Our nurturers and society increase nature's "gravity" for "falling into sex." Money and/or its equivalent is required for survival. Sex is a very saleable commodity. Because most persons "extend" their immature state of being a "love junkie," we remain driven by a need for approval. This was clearly expressed by a promiscuous patient who abhorred sex but confessed "I couldn't resist anyone who told me they loved me, even though I knew they didn't mean it." Society also rewards sex where love is limited or lacking by offering economic benefits and social and/or religious pressure to come and stay together until death do us part. Marriages of convenience are widespread! Sexual activity commonly results when a payer offers money and/or security to a needing payee; love may be of secondary importance. To the credit of human *self*-mastery, we often create love from the incentives to procreate that have been provided by nature and our nurturers. In my opinion, our establishment has yet to educate its populace to value love and institutionalize teaching the basic love (and ANWOT) skills essential for our survival. We create love through a gradual active willing process. Thus, I say "We *fall* into sex, we *crawl* into love." Love is such an important issue that I recommend you give it considerable attention and share your views with others. Our considered opinions may influence our establishment to better educate its citizens.

Summary: This stren encourages you to think more about your skill in love-making, offers a view of love to which you may compare your own, and declares that you have the capability to determine the quantity and quality of the love you create. Awareness of the LM factory within you empowers you to grow your LM skill. If you so choose to invest energy in growing this skill, you can benefit by strengthening other more basic "component" skills. The most basic skill in love-making (and ANWOT) is learning to be your own best friend, i.e., loving yourself. The self-endorsement strens provide specific direction in growing your LM factory. Other important basic skills are identified in the

Addendum and explained in this *Guide*'s strens.

Concluding learning exercises: 1. Write down your idea of love-making. And/or share this stren with another person who would be willing to discuss it with you. Express your thoughts. The goal is for you to examine your own view of LM and be able to put it into words. 2. Terrorists often claim they act for the love of their principle, usually but not always religious. Do terrorists meet your criteria of love-making? Where might they fall short?

ADDENDUM to the stren on *Your Love-making Factory*: This addendum identifies skills to grow your LM factory. As a bonus, each bit of mastery may strengthen your overall well-being. They are teachable and learnable, readily mastered step-by-step. Developing and strengthening these skills requires study and practice. I recommend studying only one or two at a time. Put each into practice. When comfortable with your understanding, go on to another. Make them available for regular review. [Note: The component skills are not ranked, just listed, although I recommend beginning with the *self*-endorsement strens.]

1. Self-endorsement, becoming your own best friend: If you were to take several random "tape recordings" of the conversation that goes on within your mind and replay them, would it sound like two good friends talking? Does it seem more like there is a terrorist(s) within your self-conversations? These strens provide effective means to become a marvelous lifelong companion to your*self*.

2. Learning from mistakes: To learn to walk, we need to overdo it, "this way," then "that way," and fall quite a few times. Children usually tolerate their mistakes better than adults. For example, a "fall" while learning to walk leads to more effort and "success." Energy is directed to learn from mistakes and make them a source of growth rather than putdowns, blaming, etc.

3. Acquiring the vocabulary of mature thinking: Words trigger patterns of thinking and action. Some simple changes in your vocabulary can promote the mature thinking that was not possible to teach or learn during your early years of development.

4. Dealing with blaming: Our natural tendency to hold someone or something the cause of our discomforts (often our *self*) usually leads to a desire to hurt or punish. Blaming wastes energy that could be used more productively. The blaming mental response is one of the easiest to identify and convert to beneficial problem-solving.

5. Using the "magical problem-solving sentence": This stren encourages use of the problem-solving approach to life's stresses rather than those that more likely lead to anxiety, depression, avoidance, and the like. **Given this situation, what is most likely to make things better for me <u>and</u> you (us <u>and</u> them), for now <u>and</u> in the future?**

6. Strengthening faith – the "yes I can" skill: Until you have some belief that you can make a real difference, you aren't likely to call on the energy available to you to make a change. This stren explains how to "borrow" some faith to get you on the track.

7. **The skill of forgiving:** Resentments and jealousy are natural, common, and rarely productive. This stren helps in recognizing this tendency and how to reclaim the energy it wastes.

8. **The "reasonable best" measure of your self-worth (avoiding perfectionism):** Unrealistic expectations are a major source of unhappiness and depression. The perfectionist is sometimes quite effective and productive but is usually among the most miserable depressed persons. This stren offers a more effective approach to evaluate your efforts and preserve your self-worth.

9. **Patience:** One of the five basic ingredients in acquiring a new skill, patience needs to be acquired, for we all enter life with the motto "I want what I want when I want it." Frequent self-endorsement for your efforts and each small step along the way create patience without the need (as one person requested) for a "crash course." Review the strens on emotional self-endorsement and secondary endorsement to grow patience.

10. **Dealing with anxiety:** Excessive anxiety, panic, and phobias are far more common than most realize. The common tendency to "what if" and anticipate the worst, usually most unlikely, possibilities rather than think "most likely" is often the source of excessive anxiety.

11. **Your value system:** Since most decisions we make are based on our beliefs and assumptions rather than scientific fact, we make more informed use of our resources when we are able to clearly identify our values. The stren, *My (your) assumptive world*, among others, encourages you to increase awareness of your own values.

12. *A newer way of thinking (ANWOT):* We are born immature and dependent. Achieving maturity, what some researchers have described as "becoming your own person" requires newer ways of thinking that often are quite contradictory to our earliest ways. The strens identified above are among others I believe to be useful components of ANWOT. They represent my attempt to develop a systemic method to teach/acquire the skills to becoming your own person, the CEO of your life. Slight modifications of a few trigger words become important substitutions that enable you to process information accurately, more so than the "native" language you acquire when you are physically and mentally immature, and likely continue to use habitually.

13. **Ultimately strengthen your skill in creating your own original strens:** The strens here offered can only be a fragment of the multitude of possible strengths that add value and meaning to your life. An important goal in developing basic skills in making your life more meaningful is to develop your capacity to create your own teaching/learning skills, ones that fit your unique life's situation. And hopefully you will create some worthy of sharing with others, adding to the general pool of strens.

----

11. <u>MY (YOUR) ASSUMPTIVE WORLD = MY (YOUR) "RELIGION"</u>

This stren encourages you to become more acquainted with *your* religion. Religion is the collection of beliefs that powerfully influence our actions. Action springs from faith in our beliefs more so than the facts we acquire from science.

This stren could just as well be called "My assumptive world." This is because each of us act in a manner that is based on the assumptions we make about our *self* and the world we live in. Science doesn't provide us sufficient facts to know our purpose in life. What is ethical and moral, what is beauty, and what is the perfect life are some of many unanswered questions. Think of all our scientific knowledge in an area bounded by a fence. What is outside the fence is taken on faith. Science continues to expand the fence that contains the facts we use in our decision-making. So much more of our actions must be based on our assumptions of what is outside the fence, what I here call "our religion". We act primarily according to our beliefs, on the "faith" we have in our assumptions. Religion is the sum total collection of our beliefs or *assumptions*. In that most of our actions are influenced by our assumptions, I believe we all are "religious"; we practice our personal often unnamed religion. Though we recognize the beliefs of most of our great religions, most persons do not faithfully put them into practice.

In my college days, I recall learning that "religion is the moral teaching of humankind." Most persons identify a specific "organized" formal religion that they ascribe to and *say* they practice. Yet, many such individuals conduct their lives so deviant from the principles of their identified religion that I question if they got the "name" correct. Others who profess no formal religion seem to subscribe quite faithfully to the moral teachings of one or more identified religions. Avowed atheists regularly act on the faith they place in their assumptions. No matter; from my point of view, everyone is "religious" because we are always acting on the basis of our particular faith, our unique set of collective assumptions. They just might not have a name for their unique personalized set of beliefs. "<u>My</u> religion" or "John's religion" may be more accurate than the broad labels we use, viz. Christian, Moslem, Jew, atheist, etc. Since our religious beliefs are so influential, wisdom suggests we familiarize ourselves with the assumptions that influence the conduct of our life.

My purpose in sharing some of my basic "religious" views or assumptions is to offer a model of one collection of important assumptions, my own. From my example, I encourage you to identify the basic assumptions by which you conduct your life. I offer "My 'religion'" as a stren for you to use in getting more acquainted with your*self and your religion*. While I believe my religion is a practical and effective one, it would be against my religion for you to blindly accept or comply with my views without critical evaluation. Rather, I would prefer to share the basic assumptive views that influence my perspective in writing the <u>Guide</u> and have this stren serve you in creating your own "My 'religion'" stren. Much of my beliefs are expressed in <u>A Newer Way of Thinking</u> - the Practical Person's Guide to Feeling Good and Doing Good. So don't be surprised if much of what I write sounds a bit duplicative.

I believe I am the "immediate" product of millions of years of evolution, and a step above the monkeys … a giant step. We used to believe we are a step below the angels. That may be true but I confess I don't even know if there are angels and, if so, whether we are very close or eons away. I humbly accept that my human capacity, while quite sufficient to serve me well in my lifetime, may be puny in the grand scheme of things. I am curious to know what came before earth and life on earth. As so many others, I assume there is a first cause or "uncaused cause" but I don't believe I have the capacity to clearly identify who or what that is and what my place is in the overall scheme. Likewise, I'd like to know if there is a hereafter and what that might be. Many people have a faith-based explanation that powerfully influences their actions. Such explanations are commonly found in most formal religions. I assume there are universal values and wisdom, and that our formal religions have identified most of them, and they share similarities far more so than differences. I believe the pervasive animosity associated with formal religions is created by our manner of thinking more so than our formal religions basic values. Our prevalent manner of thinking leads us to focus on our differences while we ignore the similarities that relate us. (This is why I believe Einstein's prophesy that we must require a newer manner of thinking is correct.)

I believe I have sufficient resources to make my life's experience beautiful, fulfilling, and productive. I have faith in my capacity to make a difference for me, and that in so doing, I'll have an impact on others and the world of which I am a part. I hold the direction of my energy to these ends to be a worthy endeavor.

My understanding of science leads me to infer I am a link in the process of evolution and that we are headed somewhere even more complex than we are now, but I personally will not experience what time ultimately brings. Consider how religions change with knowledge, for example when we believed earth was the center of the universe and the world was flat. Try to imagine the common assumptions that influenced the beliefs of cave people? Have you modified your own religious views since childhood? Yes, knowledge and "fact" does influence our views about what we don't know, but let us also graciously acknowledge <u>how</u> <u>much</u> we don't know and will not understand in our lifetime. Nevertheless, here are my important basic beliefs that I hold motivate me to use my best to do my reasonable best:

- ☻ Good deeds: – doing a deed that benefits someone(s) and/or makes the world a better place to live. The world consists of its total amount of positives and negatives. Any worthy deed adds to the total positive. ***Striving to do worthy deeds* is the simplest statement of my religion.** This is the meaning of the Jewish word "Mitzvah"

- ☻ Attaining the good life requires knowing one's *self*. The five ingredients are abundantly available: faith (I think I can!), work, patience, direction, and risk-taking.

- ☻ The Golden Rule: Treat others as I would have them treat me.

- ☻ Respect for myself and others: I strive to have tolerance for all people even if I don't agree with their assumptions.

☻ I am responsible for my actions and experience: I have been given the gift of opportunity to become my own person, to free my will from the demands of "others." I don't want to waste it. Though initially dependent on fate and circumstance, I believe as I develop physical and mental maturity I may grow my freedom from what my genes and nurturers have made of me. Such *mental* freedom is one of my most important strivings. I believe I may choose what amount of energy I invest in *self*-mastery and the payoff is invaluable.

☻ ANWOT: I continuously work to upgrade my manner of thinking to cope with the issues of modernity. I have come to believe the prescriptive, dichotomous, dependency manner of thinking inherent in our native (<u>nurtured</u>) languages is the prime source of prejudice, hatred, and wars. I believe I (we each) <u>can</u> acquire a wiser manner of thinking to consistently promote my (our) well-being.

☻ Love is an important source of energy; perhaps my (our) most important.[16]

☻ Creating and sharing love begins with loving one's self: Love like hate is a product of my manner of thinking, of my higher mental skills. I do well when I assign a high priority use of my mental energy for the manufacture of love.

☻ Become my own best friend: I will be with my*self* far more than any other. I strive to make the time I converse with myself enjoyable and meaningful.

☻ Maintain an attitude of gratitude: This wisdom is expressed in so many ways. Look at the doughnut more so than the hole. Focus on the half-full more so than the half-empty glass. Aim high but appreciate that reality often limits reaching our expectancy in spit of our reasonable best effort. [17]

☻ The Serenity prayer: I wisely create the serenity to accept the things I cannot change, the courage to change the things I can, and seek the wisdom to know the difference.

☻ The value of mistakes: Wisdom comes from mistakes; I try to accept and learn from them. Nature endowed me with tolerance for mistakes. I (we) readily accepted and learned from the many falls I required to walk. I (we) learned to abhor mistakes only by years of "training."

---

[16] "Life is short, and we have not much time to gladden the hearts of those who travel with us. Oh, be swift to love!" Sign, The Gathering Place, Hartford, CT.

[17] When we judge our worth solely by the result of our efforts we often determine and feel our self to be less than whole. The unrealistic outcome measure we are commonly taught to determine our worth need no longer be a source of self-putdowns. Carl Rogers, a therapist, put it well when he suggested that we liken our view of self-worth to a fraction in which the numerator is our expectancy and the denominator is our expectation. By sustaining a high expectancy, I aim for the best outcome; by maintaining a realistic understanding that my efforts may fall short of the desired outcome due to issues beyond my control, the resultant fraction is consistently more than "whole."

☻ Maintain high expectancy but limited expectations: *Expectancy* is the goal I strive to attain. My *expectations* conform to the reality that I have limited control of luck and circumstance, and the world often doesn't respect "fairness." Because I understand my reasonable best efforts will often result in an outcome less than the high expectancy I strive to attain, I apply the Reasonable Best <u>input</u> measure to judge my self-worth. Unlike the outcome, I am virtually always in control of my input, my ability to do my reasonable best; I thereby consistently endorse myself.[16]

☻ I am far from perfect. So it is with my own pursuit of *self*-mastery. I invest more time and energy than most because I maintain a special interest. I reserve much of me for other pursuits. I accept my limitations and expect I will continue to make unwise decisions due to my lack of perfection. I'm fond of the expression, "I waste at least half my time; I'm just not sure which half."

There are many more assumptions that contribute to how I think and feel and act. While grossly incomplete, those here identified provide the framework that permits me to fill in the spaces as the need arises to address my personal decision-making. I pursue truth and wisdom because I believe they have inherent value for creating a fulfilling life. Are you aware of the "framework" that constitutes <u>your</u> religion?

SECTION FIVE ▮

12. <u>THE "BLAMING" MENTAL RESPONSE PATTERN STREN</u> [18]

In developing <u>A PRACTICAL PERSON'S GUIDE TO FEELING GOOD AND DOING GOOD through ANWOT</u>, I have identified and labeled eight mental choices that are available to us in dealing with life's challenges. I explain each in various writings; this stren provides an easy method to identify when you are "blaming" and gets you started on how to change this nonproductive pattern.

Because the <u>blaming</u> mental response pattern (MRP) is the most widely used MRP, it accounts for more overall grief than any other pattern. It is the root of much inappropriate guilt, depression, resentment, and aggressive behavior - including prejudice. Yet, it is one of the easiest to recognize and quite amenable to change.

Blaming arises from the "fight" part of our inborn "fight or flight" pattern to manage stress. In today's world, we generally don't express our primitive tendency to physically attack what we perceive to be a problem; rather we attack with words and symbols. When we don't get our way (which is most of the time) frustration occurs and we are prone to (a) <u>blame others</u> (leading to aggression and resentments) or direct the anger inward and (b) <u>blame ourselves</u> (leading to guilt, *self* putdowns, and depression). Inappropriate aggression, resentment, and depression are unwelcome companions to most of us. Though healthy and necessary as a brief automatic response, getting stuck in blaming is a major source of day-to-day unhappiness. Prolonged blaming leads to both physical and emotional disease.

BLAMING DOES NOT LEAD TO BENEFICIAL LONG-TERM CONSEQUENCES. [Is a life-threatening situation an exception?] Blaming does provide <u>short-term</u> satisfaction to our primitive feelings of arousal. Can you think of any <u>long-term</u> benefits of blaming?

Here is a simple way to reduce much of the unwanted inappropriate aggression, resentment, and depression you carry around with you ... as clear as a blinking red light that can warn you when you are about to react in some way that compromises your happiness, your physical and emotional well-being. Apply the direction here provided with a bit of work, practice, and patience, and you will get unstuck.

---

[18] STREN - A MODEL OF A HEALTHY ATTITUDE, FEELING, BEHAVIOR, COPING SKILL OR CONCEPT THAT I CAN USE TO ENRICH MY LIFE

1. Learning starts with labeling

The first step is becoming skillful in accurately recognizing (LABELING) the response pattern to be altered. *Self*-direction requires the use of your conscious thinking; words and symbols are the handles it needs to take charge and manipulate the changes you desire.

The blaming MRP has two parts: it begins with one of the prescriptive words ... "should," "have to", "must", "ought" and ends with "and therefore, 'they', 'he', 'she', 'it' deserves punishment."
Part (1): a prescriptive word(s)
Part (2): a putdown word, symbol, or action

(a) The <u>Blaming-out</u> MRP:
"They", "he", "she", "it', "mother", "God", "the world", "the weather" did what he shouldn't have done [didn't do what he should have done] and therefore deserves punishment.

Example of blaming-out: "He shouldn't treat me that way. I ought to kick his butt." "Damn that train, it made me late again."

_____

(Fill in the favorite blaming words you direct to others)

(b) The <u>Blaming-in</u> MRP:
"I" did what I shouldn't have done [didn't do what I should have done] and therefore I deserve punishment (often a verbal attack but in the extreme, murdering one's self, i.e. suicide).

Example of blaming-in: "I should have spoken up, therefore I am ... guilty, no good, stupid, a jerk, a mouse, an asshole", and so on.

_____

(Fill in the favorite put-down words you use on your*self*)

I am primarily a ....Blamer-outer   _____

I am primarily a ....Blamer-inner   _____

I do well at both...   _____
    (Check one)

2. Practice the labeling process

Look and listen for the prescriptive blaming words -- should, have to, must, ought, need to. There are a very limited number to identify. Our response patterns are usually repeated - they have become <u>habitual</u>. Note when you are "shoulding" on others, its, or on your*self*! Each instance of blaming may be considered a negative event, causing, at least, a little bit of trauma. Repeating harmful acts without learning from them builds over time.

Each time you appropriately label the traumatic act "blaming," you slightly weaken its impact. Each recognition of "blaming" is practice towards turning a traumatic response into a learning opportunity! Regular practice will prepare your*self* to better deal with the future occurrence of the blaming.

Be prepared to <u>miss</u> more blaming responses than you label. We are not able to identify all of our blaming statements. We don't need to for regular consistent labeling of SOME blaming responses will gradually lead to easier, effortless, automatic, habitual, lessening of such blaming responses.

BLAMING WON'T BE STOPPED ALL OF A SUDDEN

Any pattern that has been repeated thousands of times will persist. Developing a new pattern will involve <u>repetition</u> and practice ... like acquiring skills of reading, of using the computer, or playing a musical instrument. Given the number of repetitions and length of time it has taken to create your present blaming patterns, how many repetitions would you guess it would take to change your blaming patterns? How many to develop a new more appropriate response?

3. Validate yourself -- let it be fun!

(a) Like working a crossword puzzle, every identification can be enjoyed. Each and every recognition of a blaming response deserves a *self* pat-on-the-back. As with airline travel points, you may need many to "cash in," yet each step along the way can bring satisfaction. The skill of *self*-validation, of enjoying each step, is also the secret of developing PATIENCE. Many persons who have great difficulty with patience ask, "Where can I take a crash course?" I know of no better way than *self*-validation, than developing a sense of satisfaction as each steppingstone is acquired along the way.

(b) CAUTION: BEWARE OF "SECONDARY BLAMING": If you apply yourself, it won't take long before you get reasonably efficient in recognizing your blaming. If you're like most, in spite of your efforts you will still find the pattern of blaming persists. And then we tell our *self* "I shouldn't have let that get by!" "I should know better by now." This is what I call "secondary blaming" - blaming our *self* for blaming our *self*. We become aware of the harm we create by putting others or our *self* down and then punish our *self* (i.e. predictably follow what the old pattern dictates) with such standard secondary blaming responses as "I'm so stupid! I should have got that last week. I could kick myself."

Do you blame yourself for making the same mistakes over and over? Can you identify what words you use when you so engage in secondary blaming? If you can, write them down.

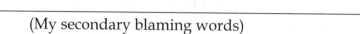

(My secondary blaming words)

Fortunately, secondary blaming is easy to deal with once we learn to recognize it by properly labeling it. Since we have been blaming our *self* so long, why would we not expect to continue to blame our *self* for some time after we become aware of continuing instances of blaming others or our *self*? Our *feelings* learn far, far slower than our *knowing* and take considerable time to "catch up."

4. Tune out the blaming MRP

Once we are able to appropriately label the blaming response, we are in a position to weaken it. We do this by learning to tune it out. It may seem strange that we have to "find something" to "lose it".   Tuning out an undesired habit is an <u>active</u> process. The value of a habitual response is that once acquired, an appropriate stressor may activate it automatically without requiring conscious effort or energy on our part. Changing habit requires conscious effort. The "tuning out" process is an action step, like erasing a misspelling - it stands in its original form, often without our being "aware of it" unless we recognize it and make the change.

Each time you recognize a "blaming" response and label it as such, stop dwelling on it, "dismiss it," pay it no attention. YOU CAN DO IT ... just as you would frequently "tune out" the radio or T.V. even though you know it is turned on. You get busy doing something else (soon to be described) and if asked, "What did the announcer say?", you may respond, "I know the T.V. was on, but I wasn't listening."

5. The creative act - the problem-solving response

In general, you would be wise to apply the problem-solving "magical sentence":
- *What can I learn from this situation that I may better deal with it for me <u>and</u> you, for now <u>and</u> the future?* This mental response will be elaborated in another stren. However, the specific appropriate action to "tune out" the blaming MRP is to direct your energy to change *prescriptive* words to *descriptive* words.

Prescriptive vocabulary: Should, can't, have to, must, ought, need to

Descriptive vocabulary: Could, I am wise when ..., I choose .., I prefer ..., What I want in the long-term is ...

Descriptive words lead to the problem-solving behavior, improving a situation. There is no "one," "ones," or "its" to be punished.   This may seem a bit simplistic, but I believe explanation of why this method is effective is quite profound. Here is my understanding.

I believe words become connected to physical responses. Words become wired to nerve patterns like the light switch on the wall is wired to a specific response. The relatively immature brain of the child can only deal with prescriptive patterns. "You must not go in the street!" "You have to go to bed." "You shouldn't have taken the candy." "You need to do what I say." And if the prescription is not followed, there usually follows some discomfort -- disaffection, scolding, spanking, or some form of putdown. Descriptive words, to the contrary, may lead to a newer way of thinking, one that asks for a creative solution to understand or resolve an issue rather than attempt to bring about change by punishment or intimidation. Whether you accept this explanation or not is OK. I do believe if you begin substituting descriptive words for the prescriptive language that is part of early training, you will find that there is change. There will be more problem-solving and less "other" and/or *self* putdowns.

6. Public affirmation: Learning occurs more surely and consistently when we are willing to generate some enthusiasm for what we are doing and then share this with appropriate significant others. As you experience the benefits of substituting descriptive words for prescriptive words, take personal responsibility for problem-solving, and become less reactive, explain it to an *other*. Periodically as you progress and get unstuck from "shoulding," sharing with enthusiasm facilitates personal commitment. Sharing also invites feedback for our critical appraisal.

Rarely will situations require an emergency response. By taking a bit of time, thinking a response through, and sharing your views with others, you are shifting the odds in the direction of making a more mature response.

SUMMARY:
1. **Learning starts with labeling.**
2. **Practice recognizing your blaming MRP.**
3. **Validate yourself with each recognition - let it be fun!**
4. **"Tune out" your blaming responses.**
5. **Substitute descriptive language for prescriptive language, problem-solving for blaming.**
6. **Share your experience with another or others.**

Follow this stren with "*Self*-Blame and Welcoming Criticism." It fits right in.

----

13. <u>THIS STREN DEALS WITH *SELF*-BLAME AND WELCOMING CRITICISM</u>

[Recognizing and managing shortcomings]

This stren explains why you get stuck in old patterns. It shows you how to resume your growth by welcoming criticism. This is one of the most important strens to feeling good and doing good. Would you practice regularly until you really get it?

"I'm so stupid. I should have learned that by now." "How could I?" "If I'm like that, I could never forgive myself." "I'm such an asshole." "Not again" "Oh, shit!" "What's the use!"

Do you find yourself uttering these phrases or some form of blaming when you discover a personal shortcoming? If so, you do what most people automatically do as their very first response to discovering a shortcoming. This wouldn't be a problem if you then went on to pick yourself up quickly. By moving on to the problem-solving method of facing and improving your many imperfections, you'll feel better <u>and</u> continue to grow.

First, recognize your usual automatic blaming response(s). By labeling it accurately, you detoxify it so that its harmful effects are considerably diminished. "That's a blaming response. I know blaming does not get me what I want in the long term. I'll challenge it or ignore it so that I don't keep dwelling on it." Even if you are a hard-working "A" student, this one step will take many repetitions over a long period.

Substitute for blaming the following problem-solving response or make up your own shorthand statement. It will become so easy and natural after a good bit of practice that you will hardly be aware that you have established a new pattern to deal with your shortcomings. The response will be condensed to a few sentences, then a word, an exclamation, and ultimately become so automatic that it will replace the old blaming pattern without conscious expenditure of valuable energy.

"As a human being, I can expect to be far from perfect. I'm going to make lots of mistakes the rest of my life. I grow most rapidly when I recognize my shortcomings, energetically face them, think them over and then do my <u>reasonable</u> best to learn from them."

While you don't remember your own attempts at walking, you have certainly observed a child learning to walk ... clumsy, swaying, too far to the left, falling, getting up, too far to the right, falling, and so on. Learning to walk <u>requires</u> many mistakes. By nature, the child doesn't condemn himself/herself. The child simply uses the last mistake to correct for the next try. Get the point - learning is built on mistakes. They are usually required. How do we get so caught up in blaming our *self* for our mistakes, as adults, when the infant seems to so productively and automatically deal with mistakes???

One of the most important growth skills I can accomplish is becoming aware of my mistakes. This allows me to take responsibility and work out a plan for change.

Therefore, every time I can identify an imperfection, my mistake, my inconsideration, I will emphatically challenge my blaming response and <u>enthusiastically</u> endorse myself for being "a wise ostrich" that takes my head out of the sand and faces the world as it really is. Avoidance brings short-term gain at the price of long-term pain.

You see, people commonly spend their lives as "love junkies," looking to others for approval as their "fix" to feel good for a little while. This is OK but it doesn't lead you to recognize your mistakes, shortcomings, and imperfections. As long as others overlook your mistake, shortcoming, or insensitivity for fear of offending you, you will go on making the same mistakes. To know you put too much salt in the soup may benefit many in the long term. Being told "what a wonderful soup-maker you are" may bring many more "too salty" soups. Any growth that you accomplish first requires recognition of what you lack.

When you accept that each time you become aware of a shortcoming, you are not "bad" or "stupid" but are indeed doing what you reasonably can to improve yourself; you deserve to say "I'm terrific!" Facing life as it is so that you can ask your*self* the magical sentence, **"What can I learn from this to become better prepared for the next time?"** is one of the most worthy acts you can make and a valid reason to endorse your*self* in the strongest way you know how.

"Congratulations to me!!! I'm doing what I reasonably can, and therefore I deserve to feel good right now for doing my reasonable best."

"Good judgment comes from experience.
And where does experience come from?
Experience comes from bad judgment."
- Mark Twain

———————

SECTION SIX ▮

14. INTRODUCTION TO THE VOCABULARY FOR <u>A</u> <u>NEWER</u> <u>WAY</u> <u>OF</u> <u>THINKING</u> (ANWOT)

The <u>Guide</u>'s first strens explain how to become one's own best friend because this skill is so basic to taking charge of our life, including feeling good and "doing good." While considering the *self*-endorsement strens, try to apply the word substitutions here briefly introduced: they powerfully update the manner we think to increase personal responsibility and *self*-mastery, and diminish dependency and blaming. Fuller explanation is provided in other vocabulary strens.

Words convey meaning. Certain words may be likened to a light switch. They are the means we may turn-*on* or *off* the path energy is processed to reach a preferred outcome. These trigger-words redirect the manner of thinking we acquire during our prolonged nurturance and dependency to alternative paths that promote *self*-mastery, responsibility, and problem-solving. The process is quite easy! **When reasonable, simply substitute the words in the right hand column for the words in the left hand column.** Most of the time, the change will "fit."

<u>Early native language dependency words</u>		<u>Substitute ANWOT *self*-mastery words</u>

dichotomous "2 *category*" words
    either ... or
	→	**analog "continuous" words**
		    both ... and

prescriptive words
    should, have to, must, ought to
	→	**descriptive words**
		    [I] prefer, choose, would like, am
		        wise when, could

dependency words
    he/ she (they, it, God) makes me ....
	→	**responsibility words**
		    I allow ....

<u>Dichotomous words</u> force our thinking into two categories: my [their/its] choices of action are "<u>*either*</u> right <u>*or*</u> wrong," "<u>*either*</u> good <u>or</u> bad," "this way <u>or</u> that." "You're <u>*either*</u> with us, <u>or</u> against us." "Do you love me <u>or</u> my sister (or her)?" *Either ... or* thinking is useful during our years of physical and mental immaturity, when our skills for processing ideas are not sufficiently developed to reflect on the complexities of our world.

Dichotomous thinking is a major source of problems in later life if we don't acquire ANWOT.

<u>Analog "continuous" words</u>, *both ... and,* more realistically convey that most of the difficult choice-making we deal with has both positives and negatives. Thus, when possible, substituting *"both ... and,"* "both this <u>and</u> that," "the positives <u>and</u> the negatives" of each alternative, will reflect a more accurate "picture" of the issue at hand. Your thinking will reflect that there are usually positives <u>and</u> negatives, "pluses <u>and</u> minuses" in the choices available to us. Rather than obsess that we *make the right choice*, we best direct our energy to *making our choice right.* So often, there are relatively equal +'s and –'s to each of our alternatives. The outcome of our choice will depend more on how we manage our choice than doing what is "right." We have no difficulty choosing between a garbage salad and a fruit salad. Choices become difficult the more balanced the alternatives. When alternatives are unequally balanced, choice-making is easy.

I find the following example helps me to understand the difference between *dichotomous* and *analog.* The old fashioned watches (and some current ones) have hands that have a continuous movement; this continuous movement is called an *analog* watch. The hands of the newer watches jump from one number to the next, from one digit to the next. It is called a *digital* watch. The hand is on <u>either</u> the 1 <u>or</u> 2 <u>or</u> 3 and so on. The connecting "in-between" is left out. Substituting *"both ... and"* for *"either ... or"* in your thinking will promote more effective management of your thinking, feelings, and actions.

<u>Prescriptive words</u> such as those in the left column are important in our early stage of development when parents, the community, and other "authorities" require that we conform to a specific pattern of behavior. If the "shoulds" are disobeyed, they usually carry a penalty imposed by the outside authority such as withholding approval, a restriction, shame, and even physical punishment. Prescriptive words convey that decision-making, personal responsibility, and mental freedom are limited, "Don't even think about it!" During our immature years, prescriptive words serve an important purpose, usually keeping us out of harms-way. They are not conducive to independent thinking. Quite the opposite, prescriptive words, when processed, mean some one, some *other*, or some *thing* is the authority whose direction "must" be unquestionably obeyed.

<u>Descriptive words</u> such as those in the right column convey a message that emphasizes problem-solving thinking and choosing among alternatives. As our brain and emotions mature, we acquire the potential to develop "response-ability," *self*-mastery. Descriptive words foster thinking that leads to independence from the more automatic habit patterns acquired over many years of practice.

Prescriptive words usually "connect" to an outcome suggesting the person, situation, group, country, religion, or thing that "did what it shouldn't have done" (or didn't do what it should have) deserves some form of punishment. *Prescriptive* words foster dependency, prejudice, blaming, resentment, and destructive aggression. Much of the *self*-blame and putdowns that result in feeling bad, inappropriate guilt, and depression are also due to prescriptive thinking. *Descriptive* words usually stimulate problem-solving thinking that invites corrective learning to seek an outcome that makes the best bargain with the situation, for now <u>and</u> in the future.

While yet working on the *becoming your own best friend* strens, also listen for the frequency you use *dichotomous* and/or *prescriptive* words. You may find it easier if you first listen for the frequency others tend to rely on the dichotomous "either...or" words and/or the prescriptive "should" words of our native language. Can you recognize that this early manner of processing information is the basis of blaming others and blaming or *guilting* our *self*? This is the source of much prejudice (pre-judged values), and the distorted thinking labeled "generalization." Examples are: A. "I don't like Bill and Joe. They each have beards. Therefore, most people who have beards are to be avoided." B. "Fido growls; therefore most dogs are dangerous."

<u>Dependency thinking</u> becomes our habitual manner of processing information throughout our first decades when we are nurtured and directed by others to conform to *their* ways. When *they* and/or the world fail to satisfy, we naturally hold *the other* responsible. Dependency thinking supports unreasonable expectations and blaming. It is also the major source of prejudice and blind obedience to authority.

<u>Responsibility words</u> such as *I allow, I permit,* stimulate problem-solving thinking and personal "response-ability" more so than the too common, virtually automatic, *Blaming Mental Response Pattern* to perceived injustice.

[Practice in these three simple word substitutions powerfully changes the manner we process information from dependency, blaming, prejudice, conflict and harmful aggression to personal responsibility, creativity, and constructive problem-solving. With repetition, the newer manner of thinking will replace the no-longer-appropriate first manner of thinking. The new processing of information will become automatic and virtually effortless. Elaboration of these important trigger-words may be found in vocabulary strens: *The Language of Self-mastery; Either...or, Both...and; Cash in Your Anger;* and throughout the <u>Guide</u>.]

----

15. THE LANGUAGE OF *SELF*-MASTERY

"... a new type of thinking is essential if mankind is to survive." ... **Einstein, anticipating the power of the bomb.** (N.Y. Times, 5/25/46) **This stren proposes the easy mental steps that update our thinking to benefit our personal well-being and that of our global community.**

Introduction

Our brain has similarities to our computer. The computer, often referred to as the "hardware," requires an Operating System (O.S.), what we call a software program, to direct the information it receives to an outcome. *Windows 3.1* was my computer's first O.S.. It has been replaced by more sophisticated operating systems. I have updated my computer with the prevalent newer operating system *Microsoft Vista*. Additional specialized software programs that more effectively process numbers, manipulate pictures, emphasize formulas or musical symbols, and/or other languages may also be added. These programs provide new paths to attain desired outcomes. Like the computer, when our brain receives data it requires an operating system to process the information to an action outcome. The O.S.s provided our brain determine the manner we think. Einstein recognized that the prevalent manner people think is not compatible with humankind's emergence into maturity. We have yet to update the O.S. of our thinking to survive the challenges of modernity. These three easy-to-do word substitutions, to be here explained, will make giant steps towards the newer way of thinking:

> **(1) Descriptive words are substituted for prescriptive words:**
>   *You should, have to, must* → *I could, would like, prefer, choose*
> **(2) Analog "continuous" words are substituted for dichotomous words:**
>   *Either ... or*   → *Both ... and*
> **(3) Personal responsibility words are substituted for dependency words:**
>   *He, she, it, they make me* → *I allow*

Who programs the manner we think, i.e. our Operating System (O.S.)?

Most of the problems of our life's experience, both personal and global, are related to our manner of thinking, the way we process information. We are our own worst enemy ... individually and globally! Einstein also told us what we must do to prevent our demise, but we have thus far largely ignored his advice. The task is quite doable and we already have the means. We only need to muster our will to take the necessary steps.

Through our early years, nature and our nurturers equip our brain with words and symbols that convey meaning. Our brain uncritically accepts the meanings we are provided to process information to action. Thus, our first O.S. is the expression of what fate and circumstance make of us. "The gift we cannot refuse" aptly describes the manner of thinking first embedded in our native language. Our early thinking has been designed to work effectively through the years that we are physically undeveloped and mentally immature. This manner of dependency thinking emphasizes whatever perspective our genes and nurturers provide. We can understand why this first O.S. is inadequate to manage the issues of our contemporary world.

Nature wires our thinking for survival. It prepares us to instinctively *fight or run* to survive. It is here-and-now oriented, impulsive, and primarily concerned about *me* (*us*), often at the expense of *not me* (*them*). Nature is amoral. *Might is right.* **Our nurturers** require us to blindly obey their authority. In our relatively civilized world, they prefer the **symbols** of power more so than direct physical aggression. We are taught to get our wants through titles, position, wealth, owning, status, "rightness," winning in competition ("beating" others), asserting God and/or the prevalent authorities are on our side, etc. However, when symbolic dominance fails, physical aggression is condoned. Immature thinking limits its conclusions to two categories such as right/wrong, good/bad, "I (we) know what is right," and seeks punishment for noncompliance. Thus, the dependency O.S. imbedded in our native language supports prejudice, hatred, intolerance, blaming others, *guilting* our *self*, and related means to engage in physical and/or mental harmful aggression.

Nature provides us baby teeth and automatically updates them with more effective replacements. It builds in clocks preset to turn-on physical maturity, such as menstruation, reproduction, and body hair. **Unlike nature's endowment of physical maturity, we receive no program that turns on mature thinking.** Rather, nature provides us "hardware," its latest most advanced brain which when mature, dwarfs any computer we create. It also provides us a beginning software program we call instinct. Thereafter, our nurturers provide us sophisticated language, humankind's product 50,000 years in the making. Mating our marvelous hardware and the sophisticated language provided by fate and circumstance, we engage in the degree of reflective thinking that makes us unique. *Reflective thinking* is the capacity of our complex brain to think about our thinking, to be conscious of our consciousness. **Reflective thinking is a gift of opportunity more so than an outright gift of mature thinking.** It is our resource to manipulate ideas, create and initiate new patterns, and most important to free our will from the directions of our early programmers. Do you see, **our first manner of processing information persists, with but minor modification … unless and/or until we update it.** Multiple studies on adult development indicate we don't take control of our thinking until our late 20's, and for many, mental freedom from what our genes and nurturers make of us is never acquired.

The manner we think powerfully influences our feelings and our actions. The dependency O.S. first acquired is the manner of processing information that may be found in every native language. This primitive O.S. is suited to our dependent, helpless, nurtured state when our brain is ill-equipped and we have little sense of "self." It becomes our main source of problems to the degree we continue to use this O.S. when we attain physical maturity. We need to update it with a newer O.S. that is more suited to the challenges of our rapidly changing contemporary world. Our recent and spreading mega-weapons of destruction demand *prevention* more so than *cure*.

A newer way of thinking = ANWOT

Updating our thinking is accomplished by substituting words that redirect information to newer pathways. I call these word-switches[19] *trigger words*. They switch the manner information is processed from one path to another. Trigger words convey meaning that influences the direction we process our thinking. They powerfully influence the action outcome of the data our brain receives. The newer trigger words may dramatically alter the action outcome. The acquisition of the newer language of *self*-mastery is attainable with maturity. Since there are a limited number of trigger words, this basic step to ANWOT is easily taught and readily learned.

Our *dependency* O.S., the software programs acquired from our genes and our nurturers, is embedded in our native language. It predictably has these four important characteristics:

1. Native language thinking is dichotomous. It categorizes information into two distinct *either…or* categories: me/not me, us/them, good/bad, right/wrong, O.K./not O.K., safe/dangerous, friend/enemy, like/dislike, and so on. Reality is distorted when thought processing is so limited. Dichotomous thinking is the basis of prejudice, intolerance, hatred, resentment, discrimination, and most of the conflict we create. The "bad" category is to be eliminated. It deserves physical and/or mental harm.

2. It is prescriptive. The orders for the conduct of our life express the perspective of nature and our nurturers. Orders are conveyed in characteristic trigger words like *should, have to, must*, and lesser used words like *demand, require*, and so on. The orders are prejudiced, i.e. *pre judged* and *pre determined*. Prescriptions commonly lead to blaming when the orders are disobeyed, followed by physical and/or mental harmful aggression. Independence, choice-making, and mental freedom are restricted.

3. It conveys our dependency on others. Our native language manner of thinking reflects the many years of immaturity and helplessness when we need to be provided for by others. This is the basis of requiring endorsement from others and remaining a love junkie when we could appropriately provide for our own basic *emotional* requirements, just as we expect and learn to take care of our own *physical* needs.

4. It is automatic. Through thousands of repetitions, as with our alphabet, the *meaning*-pathways data is processed become imperceptibly habitual and effortless. Our first manner of thinking persists within our native language virtually unchanged, unless and/or until we provide a newer way of thinking, ANWOT.

---

[19] Think of a word-switch or *trigger word* as we think of a light switch. It turns-on and/or turns-off the direction and outcome that energy flows. We merely flip the light switch and the previously placed wiring, hidden behind the wall, turns-on a predictable outcome.

Consider the characteristics of ANWOT, a newer way of thinking suited to adult maturity:

1. ANWOT is analog[20]. *Both…* and *is* substituted for *either…or.* The +'s and –'s of each choice, positives and negatives of alternative choices are processed and evaluated prior to action. Both we and they, present and the future may be considered. We greatly expand our accuracy and flexibility in processing reality. Our will is freed to mentally evaluate and rehearse infinite possible outcomes prior to directing information to action.

2. ANWOT is descriptive. The orders for the conduct of our life are *self*-initiated. Characteristic descriptive words such as *could, prefer, would like, choose, select* are trigger words that direct the processing of information to choice-making among alternatives. Descriptive trigger words turn-on creativity, initiation, and *self*-mastery. Prescriptive words such as *should, have to, must* may turn-on initiation and creativity but in the service of some "others" authority, through nature and/or our nurturers perspective.

3. ANWOT promotes *self*-mastery, mental freedom. We become our own person when we substitute *I allow* for *they (he, she, it) make me ….* We switch the dependency blaming path to a personal responsibility path. A freed will is among our most cherished goals.

4. ANWOT must be learned. Challenging an established habit requires work, patience, direction, and the application of willpower. The skills to update our thinking are easy to teach and easy to learn. Getting rid of established outdated habits is far more difficult.

Our society has yet to establish the educational resources to teach the newer way of thinking that transforms immature, dependency thinking to mature *self*-mastery personal responsibility thinking. Multiple educational resources are available for most any skill. Do you know of any courses in mature thinking? We have many institutions that teach warfare, such as the army, navy, marine, and air force academies, and multiple colleges that are military institutes. How many teaching resources can you name that specialize in peace? The payoff of ANWOT education will be huge. You are encouraged to become a part of the academy. Do you recognize that proficiency in a foreign language does not change one's dependency manner of thinking? Persons who think using their early O.S. will continue their dependency manner of thinking no matter how many foreign languages are mastered.

Additional features of our two O.S.s[21].

Our native language O.S. reflects our dependency; the ANWOT O.S. is conducive of maturity and personal mastery. Words and symbols convey meaning that triggers physical action; they have been called *our second signaling system.* They powerfully influence our primary physical signaling system such as nerves and hormones. Different trigger words initiate different actions. The specific trigger words we use determine whether we take control or allow a source outside of our *self* to push our buttons. By leaving the

---

[20] The following example helps me distinguish between analog and dichotomous. The hands of an analog watch move continuously around the dial. Nothing is missed. The hands of a digital watch jump from one number to the next missing what is in between. It is dichotomous, showing either 1 or 2 or 3 and so on.

[21] Of course we recognize that mature thinking is attained step-by-step along a continuum. We attain maturity by degree. The extremes are here emphasized to highlight differences, which may indeed by quite subtle.

prescriptive, dichotomous, dependency words placed on our control panel exposed to sources outside of our *self*, our thinking remains a servant to what nature and our nurturers have prescribed for us. Many years pass before we attain the required physical maturity and sophisticated language to take responsibility for our thinking, feelings, and actions.

Our first O.S. is most adapted to physical tangible matters such as wealth, power, recognition, appearance, and the "toys" of adult life.   The mature updated O.S. enriches the first by shifting emphasis to mental and emotional matters, viz., love, peace of mind, aesthetics, creativity, knowledge and the like. The first language must serve physical safety, our innate fight or flight response, emphasizing harmful aggression or withdrawal and the symbolic equivalents of dominance ... competition, winning, owning, controlling, etc. The second O.S. facilitates problem-solving, cooperation, sharing, developing independence as well as such skills as long-term planning, initiation, innovation, and prevention. The second language is far more adept at providing us choice among alternatives, the mental freedom we highly prize.

Prescriptive, dichotomous, and dependency trigger words belong to the first language acquired during immaturity. Descriptive, analog, personal responsibility trigger words belong to the newer ANWOT language that promotes creative choices among alternatives. When we understand these concepts and teach our self to recognize them, we may assume mastery of our *self*. Simple word substitutions upgrade our thinking to ANWOT:

Trigger words that promote dependency and blaming distinguished from *responsibility and problem-solving words (in italics)*:

Prescribing words: should, have to, must, ought, it is predetermined, I am compelled
Describing words: could, choose, am wise to, like, allow, permit, desire,
wish, prefer, decide, elect, opt, think, fancy, determine, take responsibility,
originate, cause, when this occurs then likely ...

Dichotomous words: **Either...or** --- me/not me, us/them, good/bad, right/wrong,
O.K./not O.K., safe/dangerous, friend/enemy, like dislike,
and other concepts are limited to two categories

Analog words: **Both...and** --- this and that, the positives and the negatives,
the pluses and the minuses of each alternative are considered!

Dependency words: They (he, she, they, it, God, the devil) make me ....
Responsibility words: I allow ....

These patterns of expression represent the extremes along a spectrum of motivation to act; blaming and hurting are at one end and problem-solving and helping are at the other. Blaming indicates whoever or whatever caused a situation is in need of punishment. Blaming implies the quality of badness that justifies aggression toward the blamed. Our energy is triggered to diminish that which is wrong or bad. Responsibility implies the potency to problem-solve. Responsibility = response ability. Ability is a measure of our power to respond. Descriptive words invite our skill-power to solve the problem at issue rather than the prescriptive words that lead to badness and the expression of blame. Lack of skill suggests need for education to improve our response ability. Responsibility leads to a problem-solving response. Potency is highly prized; our energy may be directed towards growth rather than destruction.

Both blaming and responsibility motivate us to act. Blaming others leads to resentment and harmful aggression. Blaming our *self* leads to guilt and depression; in the extreme, it may even lead to physical attack and suicide. Blaming may also promote avoidance and/or conformity out of fear of punishment. Taking responsibility for our *self* promotes personal growth and physical well-being. It promotes creative problem-solving for the mental satisfactions of wisdom and free choice. A happy mind influences our body to respond likewise.

While blaming is destructive, we may use it to express anger positively. Directing blame to an inappropriate action or situation (but not the person!) may mobilize our energy constructively to get rid of the "bad" or harmful act. Do you direct your anger appropriately by distinguishing between the person and the person's behavior?

Our native mental O.S. appropriately first serves our passively acquired masters; it emphasizes dependency and blind obedience to authority. Because children and animals have limited abstract reasoning ability, heeding the prescriptions of authority is usually appropriate. There is an absolute "right" in *should, have to, must, ought* ... and any alternative action is "wrong." Prescriptive words remove choice; expectations are predetermined. The primitive mind is restricted by its impulsivity and reactivity. Our native language emphasizes dominance by conflict while the ANWOT language promotes civilization. While the primitive mind deals with stress by fight or flight, a civilized mind attempts peaceful negotiation. The ANWOT O.S. strives for independence, individuality, and use of our marvelous thinking capacity for *self*-mastery of our thinking, feeling, and actions. Description words emanate from the authority of our *self* as "the describer," to select among alternatives and thus call forth choice, alternatives, and our free status. Descriptive words label the views of their creator in a manner that is not absolute. Description involves critical appraisal instead of blind obedience. The mind's work is decision-making as well as personal accountability (responsibility). Demands are not automatically regarded as *right,* to be uncritically and unalterably obeyed simply on the authority of the prescriber. Rationality and consensus are the means for critical appraisal and problem-solving action. The distinction between prescribing and describing is dramatic. Descriptive words inform more so than demand; they invite critical appraisal and are subject to interpretation, modification and *self*-management. ANWOT adds vision and greater objectivity. Of greatest importance, ANWOT promotes personal freedom. An understanding of these concepts stimulates motivation to teach our *self* to apply the trigger words of ANWOT.

We readily distinguish the implements of war from those of peace. The trigger words of immaturity and maturity are also distinct. Consider several examples of freely choosing:

Prescriptive: You [I] have to go to school. You must study.
Descriptive: If I choose to become educated, I have to study.

Prescriptive: I (you) must lose weight!
Descriptive: I'd like to lose weight; therefore, I must control my food intake.

Descriptive: Since I would like to date her, I'll have to call her and ask.
Descriptive: I believe it wise to save; therefore I must put something away.

Notice that once we our *self* make a choice, prescriptive words may be appropriate. Once we take personal control by freely choosing, by judging what is wise, then a prescriptive word automatically appears that we must obey in order to attain the goal of our own selection. The prescriptive statement that follows our own free choice is no longer expressing dependency, for I choose the goal that determines what I *must* do and I am free to alter my choice. What a difference between "I go to school because I have to" from "I go to school because I want an education." Doing out of choice stimulates motivation and cooperation.

Prescriptions often arouse our innate rebellion: "I will do the opposite of what I'm told I *have* to do; no one tells me what to do." In time, most persons recognize that such rebellion is just as dependent because the opposite action is determined by the authority's demands. However, such primitive rebellion is often our first step to realizing that we <u>can</u> challenge authority. Persons who never engage in primitive rebellion are most likely to remain stuck in whatever fate and circumstance have made of them. To what degree do you consider more so than blindly accept the dictates of outside authority? Did you (do you) "rebel" constructively or destructively?

With maturity we can not only take responsibility ("I choose to lose weight and can do it by regulating my food intake"); we can also initiate a new behavior pattern ("I'll skip lunch") that "rebels" from what we were taught. As a responsible adult, we have a choice: stay with the old habitual pattern, or consistently, actively, energetically, rationally challenge the old pattern and initiate a new one, based on the authority of our own critical appraisal. Our old patterns can be expected to persist, out of habit, unless we actively and vigorously intervene to develop new patterns of our own choosing. When we can detect our *self* engaging the trigger words of our dependency O.S., we make change possible. Simply substitute the trigger words of ANWOT to upgrade our thinking for *self*-mastery. The acquisition of this newer language of personal freedom, like the acquisition of any new language, is at first foreign and will require considerable work and patience. However, the rewards are worth the effort. Additional words and distinctions in the two languages will be presented elsewhere.

As more persons recognize the benefit and need of formal preparation in ANWOT, we can expect to see the initiation of many opportunities for education in the ANWOT language of *self*-mastery… such as book discussion groups and support groups like AA, various media such as printed material, radio, TV, the Internet and computer disks, and short courses in our accredited schools. Along with these new resources offering ANWOT, expect related programs offering the collected wisdom of those persons who have identified the bits and pieces of knowledge, which together promote our personal and community well-being, peace of mind and peace in the world, love, cooperation and the skills required for the utopian society that is in our common interest. Through ANWOT, the *mental wealth* we gain has no bounds!

SECTION SEVEN ▌

16. THE MENTAL RESPONSE CONTROL PANEL (MRCP)

This stren identifies the alternative choices available to your will as it transforms information into action. Accurate labels are our handles for thought control.

You have but eight (8) mental choices available to you to respond to any situation that you have to deal with. Most of these choices will not get you what you want in the long term; most will get you what you <u>don't</u> want. By labeling and recognizing these eight response patterns, you can make a difference by favoring the constructive responses and weakening the negative ones.

I have arbitrarily labeled the mental response choices available to us as follows:

1. Blaming-out
2. Blaming-in
3. Avoidance
4. Problem-solving
5. Self-endorsement
6. Helplessness/Hopelessness
7. Worry
8. The Mind/Body response

This stren will show you how to recognize these responses. Once you can "spot" them, you can make the substitutions that convert the harmful patterns to helpful ones. The *problem-solving* and *self-endorsement* patterns are consistently beneficial; the other six, with few exceptions, are the source of most unhappiness. Recall the basic wisdom of two great philosophers! "Happiness is a state of mind"… Peanuts (contemporary cartoon character); and "Men feel disturbed not by things, but by the views which they take of them." … Epictetus (1st century Greek). I recognize, as do you, that many individuals have wealth, status, good looks, connections, and health, yet are quite miserable. We see others lacking these assets; yet they face their life situation with enthusiasm and joy because of their mental attitude. I am not suggesting it is better to be without material assets. Given the choice, better to be (and strive to be) "a have" rather than a "have not". However, these assets do not replace the mind control you are capable of attaining that is the most significant contributor to your well-being.

Learning starts with labeling! Labels are the "handles" that allow us to direct our thinking and apply our will power to make preferred change. Some words are symbols for concepts. Concepts are mental motion pictures that serve our mind to problem solve. Labels that create accurate understanding are often all that we require to energize constructive management of an issue. I have chosen the eight labels above to reasonably include each of the mental choices available to us. Each response pattern is worthy of considerable attention. Thus, I suggest you review all eight and then consider each as an individual stren to be studied, understood, and applied over time. With practice, you will be able to integrate them into your overall "mind control" with little effort. Using the simple formulas that identify the common responses can bring dramatic results.

The most common mental response choices are the "primitive responses." These consist of *blaming-out*, *blaming-in*, and *avoidance*. They are considered primitive because they arise from our inherited biological automatic "fight or flight" instinct. The remaining mental response choices rely more on our ability to think, on the more recent to develop cortex of the central nervous system.

The two (2) Blaming Responses: Animals and primitive humans, past and present, primarily deal with danger by physical means, fight or flight. In contemporary civilization, beating on another and/or running away are frowned upon. They usually don't get us what we want and often lead to negative consequences.

Our nurturers and societal rules teach us relatively early in our lives to convert our fight energy into symbolic means of aggression. Blaming-out, i.e. blaming others, includes resentment, shunning, prejudice, labeling others "bad," "wrong," "inferior," and so on, "winning" in competition, domination via status, wealth, social, economic, and/or religious "superiority." Blaming-in is also acquired from our nurture, a modification of instinct seen almost exclusively in humans. We soon learn to redirect our aggressive fight response inward. Blaming-in includes such expressions as guilt, putdowns, self-blame, "beating on oneself," and in the extreme, suicide - "murdering oneself." Aggression directed inward is a common cause of depression. In this sense, we become our own worst enemy!

Here are some reasons why blaming is not productive:
1. It wastes valuable energy that could be directed to constructive outcomes.
2. It commonly leads to punishment more so than learning to correct the problem.
3. The assumption of "the culprit" being wrong or "bad" is often unfounded.
4. The "blamer" commonly experiences unpleasantness such as tension, resentment, bodily distress, and is subject to the many physical symptoms that result from prolonged stress.
5. Most important, it commonly leads to a similar response from the blamed: retaliation, increasing levels of destructive energy, physical and/or symbolic harm to all parties, and sometimes all-out war. We call this tit-for-tat "escalation."

The two blaming responses are among the easiest to recognize and change. Here is the formula to learn:

1. Blaming-out:
He (she/they/it) did what he should not and therefore he deserves punishment.
He (she/they/it) did not do what he should have done and therefore deserves punishment.

2. Blaming-in:
I did what I should not have done and therefore I deserve punishment.
I did not do what I should have done and therefore I deserve punishment.

Secondary blaming is a common variation of blaming-in. It is "blaming your*self* for blaming yourself." We tend to have unrealistic expectations of our ability to do what we know. Once we learn that blaming-in is to be avoided, we invariably find we continue to repeat the old habit pattern of putting our *self* down. Thereupon, we are likely to utter, "I did it again! I should have learned that by now! I'm so stupid, blaming myself again."

To diminish your blaming mental responses, first learn to recognize when you are "shoulding" on others or your*self*. Look for the prescribing words, viz. *should, have to, must, ought*. Enthusiastically endorse your*self* for spotting the blaming response in your thinking. Remind your*self* that you are now in a position to take constructive action to better your response. Substitute descriptive words such as *could, prefer, would like*. Substitute personal responsibility, "*I allow …*" rather than "*he/she/they/it makes me*." Apply the *problem-solving* mental response pattern. Periodically review the strens: The *Blaming MRP, Secondary Blaming*, and *Self-blame and Welcoming Criticism*.

3. Avoidance:
This is the *flight* part of our inherited fight/flight response. It directs us to run from harm. In animals, it is a favored means of survival. In our (relatively) civilized society, physically running away is seldom effective. First, modern technology makes it easy to find people. Second, physical life-threatening stress is uncommon whereas most persons regularly face symbolic danger and psychological stress. Thus, we learn substitute ways to "run away." [Running away to escape a mugger is better considered *problem-solving* more so than *avoidance*.]

Our mind works in many ways to avoid discomfort and/or preserve short-term pleasure at the cost of a longer-term harmful outcome. Present feelings are often more powerful than objective reason. The *Avoidance* mental response pattern is discouraged because the longer-term (and sometimes the shorter-term) outcome no longer works. Here are some readily observed avoidance patterns substituted for physically running:

procrastination: finding another activity to escape an unpleasant task
"socially running": changing jobs, spouses, friends, residences, and so on
substance abuse such as alcohol/drugs/food
telling lies – "It was my brother."
withdrawal – isolating oneself physically and/or emotionally

self-deception: the mind is so effective, deception is accepted as truth
> *denial* - "I can stop drinking whenever I choose.
> *rationalization* – "The train usually makes me late."
> "I can't help it because my biorhythms are off."
> *paranoia* – projecting our uncomfortable ideas/feelings on another
> "They don't like me because I have pimples."
> *substitution/displacement* – Angry with his boss, he kicks the dog.
> *regression* – We revert to an inappropriate pattern that previously worked
> A four year old wets himself when a new sibling gets more attention
> *physical and/or psychological "illness"* – Feigned or exaggerated physical
> and/or mental illness may excuse one from facing a stressful reality.
> Becoming Napoleon or some powerful person is more satisfying than being
> "a nobody."

Consideration of the various mental means of *self*-deception are planned to be added to the Guide at a future time. They will automatically diminish upon practice of ANWOT.

The behavioral expressions of the *avoidance response*, such as substance abuse and procrastination, are easily spotted. Patterns involving mental *self*-deception are among the most difficult because the individual believes his distorted thinking. Therefore, he lacks motivation and/or resists giving up his avoidance "defense" against discomfort. Additional interventions are required, such as love and support from others, social pressure, and/or psychological and/or religious counseling. Focusing on the positive mental responses, *problem-solving* and *self-endorsement,* often brings about the desired change without even having to directly challenge the *avoidance* mental response pattern. The negative responses tend to "melt away" as the *proble-solving* and *self-endorsement* MRP's are more regularly practiced. In addition, developing the positive responses often motivates the individual to directly attack their negative patterns.

4. Problem-solving: The most universal and effective mental resource to wisely manage our life's experience is what I call the "magical sentence" or "magical question." **Given this situation, what is most likely to get me what I want, for now and in the future, for my benefit and theirs?** While not "magic," this simple, elegant, easy to learn sentence is so effective, it works like magic. Notice, no one, no "something" is being blamed. Energy is directed to resolving and/or making the best deal with the challenging issue. With repetition, this response will become habitual and virtually automatic. It will gradually displace the negative MRP's (from disuse) even if you don't directly challenge those older patterns that no longer get you what you want. The use of the language and strens provided in this Short Course and A Newer Way of Thinking (ANWOT) will strengthen your mental problem-solving skills.

5. Self-endorsement: Endorsement means *to approve and/or support*. This "becoming your own best friend" mental skill, though vital, is one of the most neglected. Helpless at birth, we depend on others for many years. Most learn to provide for their own physical needs and would be offended if some "other" tried to attend to their feeding, dressing, bowel care and so on. Yet, I observe that those adults who regularly provide their minimum daily requirement (MDR) of *self-endorsement* are in the minority. Do you know many "love junkies" who remain dependent on others' approval for much of their *self*-worth? Who are overly sensitive to what others think? Approval is the major source of the mental energy that powers our mind. It is the basis of what we call "will power."

Unlike *blaming* that we express quite instinctively and effortlessly, we learn *self-endorsement* through willful mental action. With the intensification of approval, we generate higher levels of energy as follows:

$$approval \rightarrow endorsement \rightarrow enthusiasm \rightarrow love$$

Love is an intense affectionate concern and enthusiasm for a person and/or something. *Self-endorsement* is so critical because the ability to love another grows from our skill in loving our *self*. How do you understand "Love your neighbor as yourself"? Love is not to be confused with sex. Our sexual organs contain receptors that receive and relay messages, usually pleasurable, to older areas of the brain. The brain's pleasure area is closely related to the area that deals with aggression. Love is a willfully created and expressed activity of our latest to evolve portion of our brain, the cortex. Love and sex may go well together but they can also be quite unrelated.

Here is an easy way to evaluate if you are providing your MDR of endorsement. Imagine you could tape your thinking, the conversation in your head that you have with your*self*. Replay segments of it. Does what you hear sound as though it was a conversation between two or more best friends? No putdowns/blaming? How much endorsement, support, warmth, friendliness, problem-solving, and/or good feelings are expressed? How often do you hear, "I like what I did," "Good job," "I'm such a hot sketch," and sustained enthusiasm for your life's experience?

Secondary endorsement is an important special expression of *self-endorsement*. Since endorsement is one of our most important mental acts, we **wisely reinforce the skill of self-endorsement** by *endorsing our self for endorsing our self*. "Attaboy! (Attagirl!) Congratulations to me for remembering to endorse myself."

How can we endorse our *self* when we make a mistake, when we've used poor judgment, when "we've done wrong"? Simple! Keep in mind that the most useful way to manage a mistake is to learn from it. We already experience harm as a consequence of our error and/or misfortune. Why add to our hurt unnecessarily by blaming our *self* with various forms of putdowns? By acknowledging our shortcoming and applying the *problem-solving MRP*, we apply our energy to best deal with similar situations now and/or in the future. Blaming gets us nowhere and punishment predictably makes things worse. Stamp out blaming! Consistently endorse your*self* for recognizing and dealing with your shortcomings. I have found it helpful to recall how we learn to walk. We fall many times as we teach our self the skill of walking. As a child, we simply ask, "Did I lean too far to this or that side? What can I do to correct it?" We often show more wisdom as a child than as an adult. What causes us to become "blamer-inners?"

Among the strens in the <u>Guide</u> that deal with *self-endorsement* are: *Your love-making factory*; *Self-endorsement*; *Emotional self-endorsement*; *You Need Emotional MDRs Too*; *Curing resentment*; *How not to make mistakes*; and (The) *Reasonable best*, a measure of self-worth.

6. Hopelessness/helplessness: This "I give up" response is our most devastating because it shuts down our energy factory. It is often associated with the blaming-in MRP where it may lead to depression and significant self-harm. "Why bother," "What's the use," and similar utterances make it easy to spot. Here especially, "an ounce of prevention is worth more than a pound of cure." Prepare yourself in advance to vigorously and aggressively attack any utterance of the H/H response. Nip it early in the bud. Prepare to substitute, "It may be damn difficult, but I can do my reasonable best!" As you develop skills in the newer manner of thinking and increase your *problem-solving* and *self-endorsement* skills, the H/H response will weaken and disappear.

7. The Worry response: Anxiety attacks and phobias are common expressions of the *worry MRP*. Once you learn the formula, it is easy to recognize: We tend to "What if." We anticipate and think of the worst unlikely outcomes of a situation. Examples: *What if … the airplane engine fails … the elevator breaks down … they can't stand my pimples.* The anxiety escalates as physical "emergency response" changes occur, muscle tightness, increased heart rate, irregular breathing: "Oh my God, my heart is racing; am I having a heart attack? I can't stand it." Learn to recognize the "What if" and substitute "most likely." "Most likely … the airplane engines will get me where I want to go … I haven't heard of anyone being permanently stuck or starving in an elevator … others are more concerned about their own appearance than dwelling on my pimples." Every time you "What if," give at least equal time … think also of the very best most positive happy outcomes of a situation, even if they are as unlikely as the negative "what if's" you create. Smile and enjoy the positive "what if's." Various techniques of gradually facing the feared situation, often with some support, are very effective. So is relaxation training.

8. The Mind/Body response: The manner we think has profound influence on the way we feel and the way we act. Thinking, feelings, and actions are interconnected. This is the very reason why the newer manner of thinking is our opportunity to become director and producer of our life's experience. It is also the reason why "stinking thinking" is the source of most of our life's unhappiness.

Consider just a few of the endless list of *mind/body* responses: *skin* … rashes, hives, blushing; *vascular* … high blood pressure, heart irregularities, stroke and heart attack; *intestinal* … vomiting, diarrhea, constipation, heartburn, appetite change; *genital and urinary* … frequency, incontinence, impotence, frigidity; *muscles* … muscle contraction pain, headaches, backaches, jaw clenching, fatigue, twitches; *lungs* … rapid breathing, dizziness, asthma; *endocrine* … hormone irregularities, thyroid, obesity, sugar management, menstrual irregularities; *accidents*. There is recent evidence suggesting even cancer and infections (immunity) may be associated with our manner of thinking. Various terms have been used to identify the influence of the mind on the body such as "stress," "somatization," and "psychosomatic."

Mind/body MRPs are often difficult to recognize and to directly change. "Treatment" is often directed at the symptom, viz. aspirin for headache, dental work for teeth grinding, self-medication such as alcohol for anxiety, and so on. The newer manner of thinking, skill development in *problem-solving* and *self-endorsement* contained in The Short Course and/or A Newer Way of Thinking are especially effective means that indirectly resolve *mind/body* problems by general enhancement of your well-being.

NOTE: These eight (8) arbitrary labels of our mental response patterns will allow you to better identify your choices and wisely direct them. As you gain skill, you will begin to see combinations of your mental response choices more so than individual responses. They are not "either … or"; rather, they are "both … and, a bit of this and some of that." One MRP leads to another; they commonly work in combination; see *The MRCP, step 2*.

Summary: Our mental capacity and use of symbols enables us to join fate and circumstance as producer and director of our life's experience. We may even become the "managing partner." The mental strens or "strengths" proposed in A Newer Way of Thinking, *The Practical Persons Guide to Feeling Good and Doing Good* will "update" your manner of thinking to better deal with modernity. Understanding the Mental Response Control Panel is a powerful resource to enhance your well-being. Increase your *problem-solving* and *self-endorsement* skills as you diminish the *blaming*, *avoidance*, and other MRPs that no longer serve their original purpose, and may now cause harm. You can do it! Although the methods are easy, they require work, patience, and some direction.

----

17. THE MENTAL RESPONSE CONTROL PANEL EXERCISE, STEP 2

The *Mental Response Control Panel* stren provided labels to identify the eight choices available to your thinking as it directs information to action outcomes. Accurate identification and classification of these eight choices empowers you to freely and wisely direct your life's experience, i.e. *self*-mastery. **This stren offers animation to your labeling ability! It will enable you to see that, like elements in nature, they rarely appear in pure form; they are commonly present in combinations and continuously change.**

Given eight choices to deal with an issue, each offering some short and/or long-term satisfaction (and cost), we can understand that our thinking would seek what each has to offer. The wisdom in this stren is to convey that the eight MRCP choices are not "either/or." Thinking does not choose "either this or that," *blaming-out* or *blaming-in* or *avoidance* or *problem-solving*. Rather, we process information "both … and," "this and that," preferably a mixture of *problem-solving* and *self-endorsement* [Example: "This was sure a tough issue but I worked out a reasonable plan; congratulations to me."] more so than some combination of *blaming-in*, *helplessness/hopelessness*, and a bit of *mind/body* response. [Example: I screwed up again. Why bother. I've got such a headache."]

You make an important step to a newer way of thinking (ANWOT) as you expand your native language from "either/or" to "both ... and" thinking, emphasizing what has been described as *analog* more so than *dichotomous* processing of information. The immature undeveloped mind of the child is most suited to be taught in clearly understood "yes/no," "good/bad," "right/wrong," "O.K./not O.K." terms. After untold repetitions, such dichotomous thinking becomes habit. As a mature adult, habitual "either/or" thinking distorts our perception of the world; it contributes to becoming our own worst enemy. With eight mental response patterns, the combinations available to our thinking are virtually endless, especially when you recognize each of the MRPs may be present in varying quantity from 0% to 100%. Once you get the idea of the on-going drama and action in your mental "movie", your enlightenment and its practical benefits will really pay off. You will recognize common combinations of mental responses and redirect your mental energy to create the positive script you, as producer and director, can create.

We owe our capacity for *self*-mastery to a newer manner of thinking I call "reflective thinking." Here is an analogy that will help you understand why reflective thinking is your opportunity to add meaning to your life's experience. How much easier is it to have a mirror when you put on make-up, shave with a razor, or trim your eyebrows? Seeing your reflection allows you to make adjustments to get what you prefer. Reflective thinking is our mirror for *self*-mastery. It provides us self-consciousness. Literally, we are conscious of our consciousness. We think about our thinking. The complexity of the cortical area of the human brain and our use of symbols to create language empowers us to "see" our *self*, to manipulate our mind's activity and direct its course to serve what <u>we</u> choose, more so than what nature and instinct demand and/or what our nurturers and habit urge. **Reflective thinking** is our source of mental freedom! I call the portion of our newest to evolve brain our "freedom organ." Just as organs like the kidneys and liver have evolved to their present level of specialized function, this portion of our brain that is most recent to evolve provides us reflective thinking. It enables us to join nature and nurture as a partner in determining our destiny. As we physically mature and our nurturers teach us language and the use of symbols, we become a junior partner to fate and circumstance. The newer way of thinking (ANWOT) is the means that we may gradually become senior partner, "Chairman of the Board," "C.E.O." Recognize **your gift from nature, your "freedom cortex,"** and **your gift from your nurturers, language, and their alliance to provide** *reflective thinking.* Such enlightenment will surely arouse your passion for the opportunity of mental freedom. Enthusiasm is the most important ingredient to success in becoming master of your*self*.

Until we develop these marvelous gifts from nature and our nurturers, our thinking remains a faithful servant to instinct and habit. For nine months of our gestation period, we are clearly fated by actions totally unrelated to our doing. Fate and our genes are "boss." Helpless and immature at birth, our nurturers impose <u>their</u> stamp on our destiny. Circumstance, also beyond our control, adds its mark to what we inherit through fate. Thinking begins early but recognize that it is servant to *masters' nature* and *nurture* for many years. With luck, and the gifts of nature and nurture, we are encouraged to seek mental freedom, to become what we choose to become. But more commonly, the "establishment" directs us to blindly accept what it has determined is "good" and "right." Originality not in compliance with what our nurturers prescribe is often labeled "rebellion." It is likely to be ignored, criticized and/or result in punishment. "Masters" are prone to resist releasing their slaves. If you were unfortunate enough to be in the latter group, *self*-mastery, i.e. mental freedom, is yet available but at a greater investment of your will power. Do you see that even if fate and circumstance were unkind, you have the resource, as other unfortunates have demonstrated, to make a difference!

If you are reading this stren, you have already reached the stage in your physical and mental development that you are capable of becoming your own person. The Mental Response Control Panel (MRCP) is a powerful tool designed to assist your process of becoming master of your*self*. The MRCP stren provides the labels to identify the choices your mind makes available to you. The exercise presented in this stren will develop your skill in wisely directing those choices. Your mental strength and well-being will grow as you encourage the *problem-solving* and *self-endorsement* choices and diminish the six alternative choices that usually have negative outcomes. In short, as you recognize and develop your mental muscles of *problem-solving* and *self-endorsement*, the flab gradually withers away from disuse. Direct your mental muscles to work for you to provide wisdom, mastery, freedom, fulfillment, and enthusiasm for your life's experience.

Exercise

This skill-building exercise is simple but it requires work, patience, and some direction. It enlists your reflective-thinking-*self* to look at what your thinking is doing, i.e., to think about your thinking, to become more conscious of your consciousness.

The following pages will allow you to track your progress in increasing the degree your thinking is constructive while you diminish the harmful patterns. The first page provides the labels that enable you to recognize each of the eight choices from which you may direct your **will** to power into action your choice(s) among the alternatives. The exercise on the Score Sheet page will provide a rough estimate of the degree your thinking is helpful and/or harmful. You can monitor your progress in upgrading your thinking by repeating the exercise at intervals you choose, for example weekly or monthly. As you wisely change the frequency and combinations you apply the eight patterns, you will strengthen your will power to become the person of your choosing. I suggest keeping your exercises in a folder or binder so that you can monitor your progress in making your thinking more positive. **Make your manner of thinking your greatest and most secure asset, your *weapon for mass construction* (WMC)!**

Here is a suggestion for rating the mental response patterns (MRPs). Act as if you had a tape recording of your thinking. Isolate segments and re-play them. When you can, classify the segments. Can you identify the mental response patterns you use? Is your thinking *Problem-solving*? *Endorsing*? *Blaming*? *Worrying*? One of the other patterns? It may be easier to begin by identifying the MRPs in others. Observe their behavior. Can you think of someone who is a *blamer-outer*? A *blamer-inner*? A *worrier*? Who illustrates a combination of several mental response choices? Match yourself to others you observe and the examples soon to be provided. Which patterns (MRPs) do you emphasize?

Using the scales to rate yourself on the <u>degree</u> you employ each of the choices, you will soon recognize patterns that are characteristic of your thinking. With labeling and recognition, your reflective *self* is in a position to change the pattern. Reflective thinking is the source of will power directed by you, by <u>self-mastery</u>, more so than *master instinct* and/or *master habit.* Substitute the *problem-solving* and *endorsement* pattern each time you recognize your thinking is engaged in a negative pattern. Exercise your reflective thinking; watch and feel your mental freedom muscles grow.

Keep in mind that much of the time your thinking may not be involved in any of the identified mental response action patterns. Your thinking may simply be engaged in "pastimes," in "neutral." Also realize that each person will rate differently. That's O.K. You will attain a positive outcome by simply establishing a general pattern to prioritize your work. Support the *problem-solving* and *endorsement* Mental Response Patterns. Attack the negative patterns. Your destructive aggression and "murderous instinct" may find an appropriate outlet when directed at MRPs that no longer work, that get you what you don't want in the short and/or long-term. When engaging in the negative patterns, remember to attack the negative pattern, **<u>not</u> your self!** And, of course, endorse your*self* each time you support a positive MRP and each time you recognize and weaken a negative MRP.

This area left blank to keep the following chart on one page.

MENTAL RESPONSE ACTION CHOICE	BEHAVIORAL OR PHYSICAL OUTCOME
Blaming-out → ----- → ----- → ----- → → "He, she, they, it did what they shouldn't have done and therefore they deserve punishment.	Aggression (anger, resentment)
Blaming-in → ----- → ----- → ----- → → "I did what I shouldn't have done and therefore I am guilty and deserve punishment."	Depression (guilt, self-putdowns)
Avoidance → ----- → ----- → ----- → → Substance abuse, procrastination, withdrawal, mental self-deception (denial, lying, feigned illness, rationalization, and other means)	Short-term gain, long-term pain
Problem-solving → ----- → ----- → ----- → → "Given this situation, what is most likely to get me what I want, now and in the future, for me and you. (us and them)?"	Wise action, well-being
Self-endorsement → ----- → ----- → ----- → → "Attaboy! Attagirl! Congratulations to me for doing my reasonable best." [Congratulations to me when I recognize I'm not doing what I can.]	Energy, willpower to problem-solve, and to create and offer love
Helplessness/Hopelessness → ----- → ----- → --- "I give up!" "What's the use." "To hell with it." "Ferk it."	Apathy, depression, in extreme - suicide
Worry → ----- → ----- → ----- → → ---- → "What if …" and anticipating the worst outcome "What is going to happen?" "I can't stand it!"	Anxiety, phobias, panic, feelings of doom, physical symptoms
Mind/Body → ----- → ----- → ----- → → Mental response to stress leads to exaggerated response to physical system, viz. muscle tension, hormonal irregularity, blood pressure, etc.	Head/neck/back pain, may involve any/every organ system

THE MENTAL RESPONSE CONTROL PANEL SCORE SHEET
[Make copies so you can repeat this exercise at various intervals.]

This "well-being" exercise will help you gradually increase your use of the helpful *problem-solving* and *self-endorsement* mental response patterns and decrease the six choices that are usually harmful. Re-do the exercise at intervals you choose in order to see a trend, for example weekly or monthly. Don't be too concerned that your scoring is exact. Instead focus on increasing your **problem-solving** and **self-endorsement** MRPs and decreasing your use of the negative mental response choices. These MRPs may be used individually or combined, and in varying degrees and frequency. Like our fingerprint, they form a pattern characteristic of our personality. Unlike our finger print, we may reprogram our mental patterns to emphasize the manner of thinking that leads to *feeling good* and *doing good*.

Rate yourself **using a scale of 0-10 for** **each** **of the eight MRPs: "0" being no amount of that MRP, "10" meaning you use the maximum amount of that MRP. Total the number you assign to** problem-solving **and** self-endorsement. **Multiply by three. This is your positive score. Total the number you assign to** blaming-out, blaming-in, avoidance, helplessness/hopelessness, worry, **and the** mind/body **response. This is your negative score. The sum of the positive and negative will provide your "total" score. Mark it on the "total score" scale. Can you make the positive grow?** If your thinking is in the negative range, you would be wise to really get to work. If you're already on the positive side, wouldn't you want to add a bit more and enjoy the satisfaction of sharing your wealth?

The eight (8) Mental Response Patterns (MRPs):

	A	B
1. Blaming-in		____
2. Blaming-out		____
3. Avoidance		____
4. Problem-solving	____	
5. Self-endorsement	____	
6. Helplessness/Hopelessness		____
7. Worry		____
8. Mind/Body		____
TOTAL	____	____

SCORE: Add rating for #4 & #5   = ___ x 3 = ____ [column A]
　　　　　Add rating for #'s 1, 2, 3, 6, 7, 8.   = ____ [column B]

　　　Subtract B from A to get TOTAL SCORE = ____ [range = -60 to +60]

Are you functioning in the plus or minus range? Do you recognize characteristic patterns in others? In yourself**? Are you willing to work to increase your "well-being" score?**
Repeat this self**-evaluation from time to time. Make it a useful tool to increase your score.**

Examples of mental response patterns: see how they can change; how you can change:

1. For several years following a football injury that left him quadriplegic as a teenager, "A" was embittered, hopeless, depressed and preoccupied with dying. He blamed others and himself. One day he had an insight that changed his life. He realized that as long as he focused on what he had lost, didn't have now, or couldn't attain, he'd stay miserable. He began to focus on what he did have and what he could do. He obtained help to attend school including an aide to literally "turn the pages." He earned a degree in higher education, married and adopted a child. When I saw him, he was strikingly enthusiastic and happy. Here is a mixture of the *blaming*, *avoidance*, *helplessness/ hopelessness* response dramatically changed by *problem-solving* and *self-endorsement*.

2. "B's" parents were quite demanding and her superior performance made her their favorite among her siblings. "B" had what most persons want – smart, good looks, a good job, and recognition from her peers. Yet her perfectionism kept her quite miserable. She suffered from regular tension headaches. Whatever she did was not quite good enough, not the way it *should* be. She was what I would call a "love junkie," dependent on other's approval for her self-worth. For example, even though she had beautiful teeth, she was preoccupied with a perceived "defect" which was unnoticeable to others. She tried not to smile. Here is a mixture of *shoulding* on herself, i.e. *blaming-in*, *worry* ("what if they don't accept me"), and the *mind/body* response.

3. "C" found that a bit of alcohol before a talk relieved his anxiety. He felt (and perhaps) he did better. Similarly, he found relief from marital stress. In time alcohol was like a "best friend." It gave him immediate comfort, was uncritical and readily available. You can imagine how the short-term gain brought increasing longer-term pain. When those who cared urged him to abandon his "friend," he became resentful and adamantly denied his growing dependence: "I can stop anytime I want!" As his work and marriage deteriorated, he was given an ultimatum, "get help or else!" While at first reluctant, his resistance to AA gradually changed to enthusiasm. He acquired the wisdom others offered. His newer manner of thinking led to one of his greatest satisfactions, helping others by doing *12th step work* (mentoring others). What MRP's can you identify?

4. "D" had such panic episodes she came to avoid most situations. She could not take her graduate exams, refused to drive an automobile, and her "what if" thinking regularly pictured the worst of all outcomes. With encouragement and support, she step-by-step confronted her fears, for example, slowly expanding her boundaries, including driving. As the "what iffing" changed to "most likely" and she grew confident, she was able to take and pass her graduate exams. She established a more wholesome life style. Can you recognize the change in her mental response patterns?

5. "E" was adopted when her new dad wanted a daughter rather than his biologic son. Her presence was a rose to dad, a thorn to mom. Life for E became quite difficult when several years after her adoption, dad died. The balance of "favored" (dad) and "reject" (mom) was suddenly "reject." E was no longer the prankish spoiled child; she quickly became a hellion. All that goes with blaming-out, especially lack of consideration for

others bloomed. As she later expressed, "Better to be rejected for what you do than what you are. You can always change what you do; you can't change what you are." What MRP's can you identify? Could self-endorsement skills make a difference?

SECTION EIGHT ▌

18. LIFE'S WISDOM

This stren is a collection of practical assumptions people commonly arrive at through experience and reflection. To them, I add my own condensed list.

After years of therapy, patients often come to certain basic assumptions. A teacher of therapists* has identified common ideas people arrive at after wrestling with life's conflicts. These same conclusions are found in "rules of living" laid down by poets and philosophers from the earliest times. They are bits and pieces of mental "strengths," the wisdom(s) which harmoniously joined, permit a style of living more in keeping with reality. Are they similar to your own?

As expressed by patients:
1. All people have problems and I know now that mine are no worse than anybody else's.
2. I realize I considered my symptoms a sign of weakness. I realize they aren't. I don't pay attention to them and they pass. They aren't such a big deal now.
3. One of the big problems I had was considering myself the center of the universe. It now isn't so important for me to feel so important.
4. I was so full of guilt I felt I would bust. When I talked things out, I realized my standards were a lot stricter than those of other people. As a matter of fact, I would purposely do things to prove I was bad; now I don't have to.
5. The price I would pay for my indulgences was just too high. So I don't burn the world up! So I don't get as much of a bang out of doing ridiculous things! The quietness I feel more than compensates for the high life I was leading.
6. Why knock yourself out climbing on top of the heap? You're nowhere when you get there. You kill yourself trying. I was so ambitious and perfectionistic that I had no time for living. Now I try to find pleasure in little things, and it works.
7. I don't have to blame my parents anymore for my troubles; whatever happened happened. Why should I let the past poison my present life? I feel I can live now for what life has to offer me right now.
8. I used to torture myself about the future. Worry about it so much I couldn't enjoy anything. I knew I was silly, but I couldn't stop. Now I just don't care. I do the best I can now and I know the future will happen as it will happen no matter how much I worry about it. I take things as they come.

*Extracted from <u>The Technique of Psychotherapy</u>, Lewis R. Wolberg, M.D., 1977

I wish to add several "wisdoms" to the above that I have found useful for myself. Here are 10 basic ones :

1. Just as I've come to accept I am responsible to provide for my physical needs, I am responsible for my mental and emotional well-being.
2. I work to become and remain my own best friend. I live with myself far more than all others combined.
3. I best maintain mental and emotional well-being by directing my thinking to what I have attained, what I have now, and what I may yet achieve. [I create unnecessary upset to the degree that I <u>excessively</u> dwell on what I have lost, what I don't have, what I may never attain.]
4. I have learned and believe that the most common basic ingredient to success, whatever my endeavor, is **chronic enthusiasm.**
5. Perhaps the most powerful words uttered: "Forgive them, they know not what they do." Resentment and revenge too often result in mutual hurt and escalation of problems, in "lose/lose" outcomes in the short and/or long term.
6. Actions are largely based on values. Virtually every religion accepts some version of the Golden Rule; it's a good beginning for a universal value system. "Do unto others as I would have them do unto me," or "Love thy neighbor as thyself." [What does this say about self-love?   What are your views about self-love?]
7. I <u>work</u> to accept what I can't change, to change what I can.
8. I welcome love from others and know it's worth working for; I try not to depend on it by regularly providing myself my minimum daily requirement (MDR) of self-endorsement.
9. Express love as a gift, not as something given to get.
10. I have created faith that what I do <u>can</u> make a difference! "I can if I think I can."

I value these additional bits of wisdom:
11. My interpretation of events is more critical than the event itself. Maturing to an interpretive creature, I assume major responsibility for my life's experience.
12. "Know thyself" -- the basic tenet of Socrates, Christ, Freud, and many others. We both guide, and are guided, by our views. [Science provides facts; we create belief. Because religion is the sum total of our assumptions, all people are religious. Are you familiar with your religion?]
13. My <u>three</u> masters are those physical forces outside me, those physical forces inside me, and the mental forces I create. Thinking is my source of *self*-mastery. [Helpful vocabulary words explained in the glossary: exogenous, endogenous, mentogenous (outside, internal, and mental directions)]
14. The greater control I exercise over my thinking, the greater my will power to influence how I feel and how I act.
15. Freedom is universally cherished. Mental freedom requires skill in challenging instinct and habit, our nature and nurturers, fate and circumstance.
16. *Self*-mastery is mental freedom; it is best exercised with wisdom. The wise expression of *self*-mastery requires a newer way of thinking (ANWOT).
17. When possible, I substitute descriptive words for prescriptive words, i.e. substitute "could," "choose," "would like," "prefer" and related **responsibility** words for

"should," "must," "ought," "have to," and related *blaming* words.

18. When possible, I substitute "both … and" for "either … or", i.e. "continuous" words for "dichotomous" words. Dichotomous (limited to two sides) are "either … <u>or</u>" words such as "right/wrong," "good/bad," "us/them," "black/white." Most situations contain both pluses <u>and</u> minuses.

19. I have identified eight mental response choices available to me. [See *The Mental Response Control panel* stren.] I try to regularly apply the most useful one, the "magical" problem-solving response: "What is most likely to get me what I want, now <u>and</u> in the future?" With rare exception, this includes an "other" also getting what benefits *he, she, they,* and/or *it*.

20. I try to recognize and stop the unhelpful mental responses, the most common being blaming others or myself, avoidance and procrastination.

21. Though less common among the eight mental response choices, I especially refrain from the most devastating one, the helpless/hopeless response. I recognize the H/H response shuts down my energy factory.

22. Peace of mind requires work, then practice, practice, and more practice! Though quite attainable, there aren't many short-cuts.

23. Peace of mind and well-being may be created with five ingredients: the simple faith that I can make a difference, work, patience, a bit of direction, and risk-taking (i.e. the willingness to challenge instinct and habit). It does <u>not</u> require unusual intelligence, material wealth, status, "connections," membership in a specific group, or even good physical health, although given the choice, have them rather than not. Magic isn't needed!

24. Most help is *self*-help … often with and through others.

25. "We stand on the shoulders of the giants who preceded us." We are what we are because of other people. They provide wisdom and direction. I try to recognize my support people and role models, and willingly seek the help and knowledge others have to offer.

26. As our organs are a part of, and essential for proper function of our body, I recognize that each of us, similarly, is an integral part of a larger system. Contribute to its well-being rather than hurt it.

27. In today's world, emergency situations are rare. I try to *act* rather than *react*, to manage adversity emphasizing reason more so than instinct.

28. Others have shown effective persons often demonstrate these three qualities:
    a. *Accurate empathy*: the ability to understand the other's feelings and convey it
    b. *Unconditional positive regard*: respect for the person, not necessarily the person's view(s)
    c. *Congruence*: consistently being the same recognized person; not warm one day, cold the next.

29. *Good aggression* is the direction of our energy to benefit others as well as our *self*; therefore I seek "win/win" rather than "win/lose" outcomes.

30. I regularly substitute the "reasonable best" measure of my self-worth for the "absolute best" measure many persons use. "Given my limitations of time, skill, and energy, I endorse myself for doing my <u>reasonable</u> best. I can do my reasonable best virtually all the time." See the *Reasonable Best test* stren, pp. 21-23.

31. I know it is human to make mistakes. By doing my reasonable best to recognize and correct them, I consistently endorse (not beat on) myself.
32. I set ambitious goals and work hard, but accept that I commonly won't achieve them.
33. To lessen disappointment, I maintain expectations <u>only</u> about what <u>I</u> control (my thinking); I maintain high expectancy, but no expectations about what I don't control, e.g. how others think and act. I energetically work to bring out the best in what I don't control.
34. By facing and accepting my limitations, I create an attitude of gratitude, and respect what I have now as precious. Plato summed up his life's wisdom in two words – "Practice dying."
35. Criticism is best offered out of concern, not as a putdown.
36. I try to welcome critical comments; I know I'm not required to agree with them. Flattery feels good but I'm more likely to learn from criticism. [Even when the criticism is ill-intended, often I still learn!]
37. Choices are difficult because they involve pluses and/or minuses in each alternative. When faced with difficult choices, I think more of making my choice right than making the right choice.
38. The attainment of wisdom is a life-long quest. The thought that I may be a link to share and/or pass on any wisdom to the next generation is itself fulfilling.

What important assumptions are on *your* list of "life's wisdom?" How would you add to, subtract from, or modify this list?

----

19. TEN WORTHWHILE "ADDICTIONS"

For most people, "addiction" is "a bad habit, something to get rid of." This stren addresses addictions that are worthy to cultivate, that will greatly enhance the quality of your life.

"Addiction" commonly means we acquire an experience so powerful that it wants to be repeated; and it occurs automatically, with little or no effort, and with such force that it requires great will power to resist. Sometimes it includes physical effects. The alcohol addict may experience irritability, shaking, see imaginary things, and have convulsions. The heroin addict who fails to supply his acquired drug habit experiences muscle and intestinal cramps, nausea, diarrhea, restlessness, and sometimes spontaneous orgasm which is described as "draining," weakening and unpleasant. The addict may experience little or no noticed physical response but have severe mental and/or behavioral effects such as the craving, preoccupation with specific thoughts and/or performance of specific acts. Consider what occurs with the gambler, smoker, the "food-aholic," the praying of the "religious addict," the guilt and/or resentment of the "blamer," the perfectionist, and the more gender stereotyped "addictions," viz., preoccupation with sports or the "appearance addict" whose discomfort grows with their perceived need for makeup, a regular visit to the hairdresser, and/or concern about their body size and shape. I recall one woman who was so constantly preoccupied that her teeth were so ugly (they were actually quite perfect) that she persistently worried and refused to smile in public. **Addictions have powerful physical, mental, and/or behavioral components.**

Addictions need not be negative! Indeed, **addictions can be beneficial, even life-saving.** Consider one simple acquired habit: looking both ways before crossing the street. It protects our life and warns us with a bit of discomfort should we fail to exercise this action. Positive addictions enhance our well-being and often prevent us from acting in a nonproductive manner!

Positive addictions are very important. Because they occur and reoccur relatively automatically with little or no effort, they spare our energy for new activity, new enthusiasms. Positive addictions ensure the consistent regulation of our mental and behavior actions just as our heart and liver orderly manage our physical sustenance. Most can readily be acquired and they remain faithful to their purpose, once established. Wouldn't you like to have an assistant helper, who will quite merrily work on your behalf, for your health, happiness, and well-being, with little or no demand for payment?

I have come to realize that positive addictions are so useful that I have identified some of the ones I consider most worthy of cultivation. Each is readily teachable and learnable, as explained in the Guide's strens.   You already have many positive addictions. I have prepared this list for your consideration:

1. Faith that my efforts count: the belief that I can become responsible for my*self*. The process of taking charge of my life's experience, what has been called "becoming our own person," begins with the faith that what I do does matter. Absent this belief, there is a tendency to apathy and/or to blame "others" for not providing what we can do for ourself. Science does not bridge the leap to faith. However, the mere observation that many others, including those with the most severe limitations, make their life fulfilling is one inspiration to acquire the required faith to start with the premise, **"Yes, I can!** I think I can, I think I can, I think I can." Recall the marvelous child's story, *The Little Engine that Could.*

2. Self-endorsement: skill in habitually conversing with our self as one's best friend would with another. Just as we have a minimum daily requirement (MDR) for vitamins and physical nourishment, we have a MDR for mental endorsement. As adults, we don't expect others to support us, feed us, clean us, attend to our bowel needs; yet, we commonly neglect to teach ourselves to regularly provide our MDR of mental and emotional endorsement. The skills of self-endorsement are presented in many strens throughout this Guide.

3. Loving, friendship: by filling our needs through self-endorsement, we "spill over" love and share with others. Love is a willing "gift" that is offered without strings or demands of "repayment."   Giving to get is too often an act leading to disappointment. The act of giving of ourselves, what we have created, is inherently *self*-satisfying. In cultivating meaningful relationships, we also expand the opportunity for our personal growth and knowledge that comes with sharing. Consider the stren, *Your Love-making factory* and related strens there indicated.

4. Chronic enthusiasm: the habitual use of our energy for rewarding action.
Whatever the goal, success is most likely when pursued with chronic enthusiasm.
Persons who consistently feel good and do good seem to regularly generate
enthusiasm by rewarding themselves for exercising effort towards a desired goal.

5. Belonging: Just as we consist of many internal organs that make us whole, we
are also a part of the greater community within which we thrive. Developing the
habit of "doing good," in addition to "feeling good" sustains the harmony we may
attain through our communal interest.

**6. Wisdom: the constructive application of abstract thinking, reason, probability,
and the knowledge acquired through the past and current experience of "others."**
An addiction to seeking wisdom is the key ingredient to enhance the well-being
of ourselves <u>and</u> the community to which we are a part. Too often, the will
power of *self*-mastery is harmful when applied without wise direction. *Self*-mastery
+ ANWOT + wisdom ⇒ peace of mind, peace for humankind.

7. Work: the application of our energy to attain a desired goal. Work is the
path that enables us to fulfill our needs and wants. It can be very fulfilling as we
experience a "good tired." We are not inherently lazy; we willingly work hard when
we foresee its productive outcome. Freud concluded the two human endeavors
that make for a satisfying life are "lieben und arbeiten," to love and be industrious.
What a marvelous combination when we learn to love our work!

**8. ANWOT: acquiring the words, ideas, and assumptions of the new way of
thinking (ANWOT) compatible with becoming one's own person.** The "native"
language we acquire through repetition, when our mind is undeveloped and our
body is immature, addicts us to a childlike manner of thinking, and thereby feeling
and acting. It shapes our thinking to have unrealistic expectations from "others,"
overdo blame and guilt, and remain dependent on the "prescriptive" and "either
… or" processing of information that sustains the prejudices of our upbringing.
ANWOT is the readily taught and learned substitution of newer words and
concepts that promote rational problem-solving more so than reaction and action
through instinct and habit. Our early manner of thinking emphasizes trial-and-
error learning from mistakes and role-modeling. We can no longer afford to learn
from nuclear mistakes in our new age of destructive power. ANWOT emphasizes
prevention, "no-trial learning" through forethought and rational mental processing
of alternatives <u>before</u> action is taken. While we enjoy our physical freedom, most
people are unaware of the degree we remain mentally addicted to the perspectives
of our genes and nurturers … not until their second or third decade as they acquire
physical and mental maturity. The focus of this <u>Guide's</u> collection of strens is
addiction to a manner of thinking that promotes *feeling good* and *doing good*.

**9. Life style, nutrition, and exercise: promoting the habits of daily living that
grow and maintain our physical well-being.** The skills regarding nutrition and
life style are now widely promoted while the benefits of certain life styles are
increasingly being identified. Acquiring ANWOT strengthens our will power to

more regularly do what we understand to be in our best long-term interests.

10. Mental growth, education: Addicting ourselves to the chronic pursuit of practical knowledge and its beneficial application throughout our life, and especially in our later years when our physical resources are declining. Habitually exercising our mind is equally and perhaps more important than the usual measures we take to promote our physical health.

I have found these ten addictions so useful that while I'm at it, I will add another ten:

11. Risk-taking: the willingness to let go of established patterns to make way for newer, more appropriate and effective ones. How we wish to cling onto what has worked in the past, even when we recognize that it is no longer currently effective or appropriate. Necessarily, "old friends" die and sometimes it is our task to willingly aid in their passing. You can understand why "risk-taking" is a fearful ingredient of change, yet it is essential for growth. I like the analogy provided by Gail Sheehy in Passages: like the crustacean, we must allow ourselves to become vulnerable as the old shell is shed to make room for our new place in life.

12. Optimism: anticipating the positive outcome that we may experience from our participation in life's activities. The use of forethought, fantasy, and mental creation of positive possibilities enhances our energy and directs it to constructive use. It is virtually the opposite of "worry," dwelling on the worst, usually unlikely outcome of our life experiences. Too often we waste our energy in worry, creating unnecessary anxiety, phobias, and the like, when we would be wiser to "optimize." While objectively processing the data of our life's experience, "optimizing" can be very productive and certainly a better choice than "worry" when we do stray from reality.

14. Patience: the ability to forgo satisfaction now by mentally gratifying our *self* now to attain greater benefits (or avoid pain) later. We are all born wanting what we want "now!" Emphasis has been growing on "faster!" We are initially addicted to impulse, to "sell our soul" without forethought until we acquire effective means of thinking. Patience is one of the more difficult addictions to acquire; unfortunately there is no "crash course." It is surely acquired with skill in self-endorsement.

15. An attitude of gratitude: acquiring the skill to habitually appreciate what we have attained, what we have available to us now, and what we may attain in the future creates a state of mind that leads to feeling good and doing good. Alcoholics Anonymous is a staunch advocate of this important addiction.

16. The three "success" skills: accurate empathy, unconditional positive regard, and congruence. Research and observation show that these qualities routinely lead to successful outcomes in both individuals and programs that exhibit them.
   a. **accurate empathy**: the ability to empathetically experience the perspective of the "other" and convey that we understand (not necessarily agree)
   b. **unconditional positive regard**: experiencing and conveying respect and

concern for the well-being of the "other" (not necessarily the "others" ideas and/or actions)

c. **congruence**: being consistent and reliably conveying the above, not so one day and quite different the next.

17. Music: song, dance, movement: rhythm and engaging the symbols of music may enrich our mind, provide entertainment, influence our mood, invigorate thinking, and promote cooperation and mutual understanding through shared participation. The physical benefits are evident. Enriching activity tends to "squeeze out" negative preoccupation. Such activity is readily and freely available, irrespective of status, and usually harmless to others.

18. Hobbies: in addition to the pleasure innate in their pursuit, the acquisition of chronic enthusiasms promotes and sustains our vigor. David Starr Jordan, first president of Stanford University, wrote a book extolling the desirability of acquiring multiple interests in our youth, more than we can possibly fulfill, so that they sustain us when we may have difficulty generating new enthusiasms.

19. The "reasonable best" measure of self-endorsement: given our limited time and energy, habitually complimenting ourselves when we do what we <u>reasonably</u> can to "do good." We frequently don't succeed in achieving what we prefer, often due to circumstances beyond our control. Commonly, we have other more important priorities, and of course because we are human, we are certain to make many mistakes. Perfectionists make themselves unnecessarily miserable due to their unreasonable expectations. Notice the "reasonable best" measure is an "input measure" that is within our control, unlike the "outcome measure" more commonly and unwisely used to judge oneself.

20. The Magical Sentence: "Given this situation, what is most likely to get me (and you) what is beneficial in the long-term as well as the short-term?" Dealing with life's challenges using rational problem-solving is usually more productive than the automatic responses we acquire through instinct and/or habit. This powerful sentence promotes the mental "habit" of no-trial learning through reason in dealing with life's challenges. Learning to habitually guide our actions by this sentence is most likely to promote wise productive and beneficial outcomes to our action. While not "magic," it works so well, it is magical.

What positive addictions do you have? Are there some you'd like to develop? What would you add (or subtract) from my list? Do you realize that you can readily enhance and/or add to your positive addictions? **What are you willing to do about positive addictions that you might want for yourself?**

While I am "on a roll," I will share my view of one more positive addiction because of its universal interest. My assumptions re its positive addictive qualities are clearly open to alternative opinion.

21. **Actively and regularly experiencing sexual gratification:** Sexual activity has many positive and negative aspects. Here I explain why I include regular sexual gratification in my list of positive addictions that are worth cultivating:

   a. **Sexual activity is generally considered our most pleasurable natural physical experience.** Perhaps sex is so paramount because survival of the species depends on it. Animals seem chemically "required" to risk their lives to perform the rituals of reproduction. While we are also powerfully driven, we do have choice. Instinct, pleasure, curiosity, culture, parental and/or other social interests powerfully motivate sexual activity. Sexual gratification brings both discharge of "sexual tension" and intense pleasure. Sexual tension builds up with thoughts of re-experiencing pleasure, and cyclic interest is established.

   b. **Sexual interest occurs throughout the major part of our life.** Sexual activity intensifies at puberty when nature's biological clock begins to audibly tick. It does so through many decades until gradual decline in performance, and sometimes interest, with aging. This may be due to the direct "wearing out" of our sex-related biology, or the indirect effects of other physical and psychological changes.

   c. **Sexual "need" is 100% satisfiable.** Self-satisfaction is readily available, free of charge, irrespective of status, race, religion, creed, etc. The preponderance of evidence is that self-gratification is not harmful to oneself and need not involve an "other." Physically, our sexual organs are <u>receptors</u> of physical stimulation; they <u>receive</u> information, irrespective of who or what is providing it. Thus, sexual gratification is available at one's will, without an "other." It has been said, the only time you can be certain of the sincerity of your partner is when it is yourself. Self-stimulation is rarely associated with harm to oneself or others.

   d. Observation and studies indicate that persons regularly experiencing sexual gratification enjoy greater well-being and longevity.

   e. Sexual activity with an "other" commonly fosters related positive experiences: social sharing, intimacy, companionship, love, cooperation, and procreation.

   f. Suppression of sexual gratification commonly leads to deviant forms of expression that may be harmful.

Humankind are "interpretive" creatures. What has been said above about the positive aspects of sexual addiction may be reversed by one's personal assumptive views, cultural and religious beliefs. Sexual activity can be a source of significant harm when unwisely expressed. There are clearly consequences that can turn a positive addiction into a negative one. Appropriate, honest information and preparation increase one's likelihood of making sexual pleasure a positive addiction.

RECOGNIZE, PRACTICE, AND ENJOY YOUR POSITIVE ADDICTIONS

EVALUATION: A NEWER WAY OF THINKING

The Educational Community strives to continually improve the materials that you receive. Your input re any portion of this request for critical comments is appreciated. Reach us by mail or the Internet [www.anwot.org].

1.   Approximately what percentage of the materials have you read?

2.   Which strens have you found most useful? Why?

3.   Which strens have you found least useful? Why?

4.   What would you change? Add? Omit?

5.   Would you write strens you consider most helpful in your thinking? [The E.C. welcomes receiving copies of any such strens. If the program grows we'd hope to pay for any stren selected to distribute as part of the basic collection. However, you best expect to receive the greater benefit from the insight you will gain by formulating in writing the strengths that are most important to you.]

6.   Can you identify any way the <u>Guide</u> has been helpful and/or harmful to you?

7.   Do you feel the strens have helped you become more your own person? Comments appreciated.

8.   Do you have interest in starting a discussion group or a local chapter of "A Newer Way of Thinking"? Our materials and help are free if used *not for profit*.

9.   The purpose of the <u>Guide</u> is to strengthen your thinking in several ways: (a) to provide the skills to think independent of what fate and circumstance demand and thereafter to wisely direct your thinking to constructive outcomes, (b) to feel good and do good by becoming a better friend to your*self*, and most important (c) to participate as a member of the larger community as a warrior for peace of mind, peace for humankind. Do you believe this educational approach has assisted you in strengthening these goals? Could do so for others?

10.   Our internet site provides the Educational Community the means to disseminate strens at no cost to any person in the world. Given our mission, "peace of mind, peace for humankind," what suggestions can you offer to further this goal?

EPILOG

It seems to me that nature works backwards in that it first requires that we take the test and then we may acquire the answers from our mistakes. Wisdom grows from mistakes. I've made my share and I suspect you have made a few. However, in the course of completing most of my life journey, I have grown quite mentally wealthy. <u>The Short Course to Mental Wealth</u> is my attempt to stimulate you to continue on to even greater wealth than here offered. Most of the wisdom here contained has to do with *becoming your own best friend*, lifelong. It is the prerequisite skill to the greater challenge of creating peace in the world. I believe each of our efforts contribute to making the world a kinder gentler place. World peace is quite attainable and our wisest choice among the alternatives. Thus, I urge you to proceed to the more challenging course, <u>A Newer Way of Thinking</u>, especially the section entitled "Good Aggression." You have permission to make copies of any or all of the materials and offer them to others with but one condition – if they are passed on for material profit, you are required to obtain written approval of The Educational Community, Inc. through its Internet site, www.anwot.org. The full course is a comprehensive proposal to spread the peace we universally desire. It is available **free** on the Internet site. You may read it on the screen and/or down-load it to make a hard copy for more convenient reading. From the Internet site, you can also order a CD of the full course for the cost of mailing. They make nice gifts; you may make multiple copies to freely distribute. As of this writing, I am seeking a publisher to make the full course available in print. While I have limited control of the commercial printer's cost or retailers profit, I pledge that I have no profit motive save whatever funds that may be generated will be used by the non-profit corporation, The Educational Community, Inc. to further its purpose to spread a newer way of thinking.

<u>PAY IT FORWARD</u>

Become a force to spread ANWOT and promote three goals – *becoming one's own best friend, becoming one's own person,* and *contributing to world peace.* If you would like a loved one or friend to benefit from the <u>Short Course</u>, please offer to pay that person(s) to take the course. Offer them a material benefit that you will pay when they notify you they have completed the <u>Short Course</u>. Let them know it is FREE on the Internet or send them a published copy. I recommend offering a "gift" such as ten dollars, a treat to their favorite restaurant, or some material reward you know your loved one would like.

Congratulations for reaching this page in the <u>Short Course</u>. As you apply the wisdoms offered, your mental wealth will keep on growing; there's no limit. I wish you even greater mental wealth and that you reap the joy of giving it away!

Donald Pet

"Everything is changed. We shall require a substantially new manner of thinking if mankind is to survive."... Albert Einstein on conceiving the $E=mc^2$ formula that led to the creation of our new atomic era including weapons with hardly imaginable destructive power.

BONUS SECTION

PREVIEW OF <u>A NEWER WAY OF THINKING</u>

Our world faces a crisis as yet unperceived by those possessing power to make great decisions for good or evil. The unleashed power of the atom has changed everything save our modes of thinking and we thus drift toward unparalleled catastrophe. .... a new type of thinking is essential if mankind is to survive and move toward higher levels. [22]   *... Einstein*

This bonus section is provided to inspire you to continue your graduate studies in well-being. <u>The Short Course to Mental Wealth</u> provides the important mental skills that enable you to become your own best friend; it introduces you to the language and wisdoms that are required to become your own genie. I hope you have enjoyed and profited from it. Excerpts from the more challenging book, <u>A Newer Way of Thinking</u>, are here provided to serve as the aroma to entice you to partake in the full meal. More than the "what to do directions" of <u>The Short Course</u>, the full course explains why destructive aggression defines our history and will prevent us from continuing to make history ... unless we heed Einstein's advice. It provides an understanding of the way we think so that ordinary persons can become the architects and engineers who will complete the road to civility that is but partially attained. Shown the way, the masses will gladly follow. Popularizing the newer way of thinking is our best hope to prevent our self-destruction and to use our new knowledge to further our well-being.

"Our world is nearing an end!" "Apocalypse is near!" Such warnings, long uttered by some extreme religious groups, are regarded by most as "wacko." They are more difficult to ignore now that these warnings are supported by our most respected scientists. The Bulletin of the Atomic Scientists, including 18 Nobel Laureates, concludes it is only a matter of time before the release of our newer weapons of mass destruction will create Armageddon. In 1947 they created a "Doomsday Clock" to warn us of the world's vulnerability to nuclear weapons. In 2007, they moved the hands forward two minutes, to five minutes to midnight (Doomsday). It had been unchanged since February, 2002. Their action reflects the growing risk, including nuclear ambitions of multiple countries, unsecured nuclear materials, the continuing "launch-ready" status of 2,000 of the 25,000 nuclear warheads held by the U.S. and Russia, escalating terrorism, and new pressure to expand nuclear power. (Bulletin of the Atomic Scientists; www.theBulletin.org)

---

[22] The New York Times; May 25, 1946.

Most knowledgeable persons agree that the threat of nuclear holocaust is the greatest immediate threat to humanity, exceeding our valid concerns about global warming, the environment, and hunger. The clock is tick, tick, ticking away.

It takes minutes to unleash a nuclear arsenal. We can expect little or no warning and there is no defense. The number of persons who can release nuclear weapons by the push of a button or the utterance of a word is growing. Experts tell us there is as much chance for Star Wars from the misinterpretation of a perceived "enemy" action or a mechanical malfunction as an actual declaration of war. This cancer, nuclear holocaust, requires swift action because it is so virulent that it is rapidly fatal, targets loved ones, attacks people of all ages, and its precancerous condition is prone to rapidly metastasize. Most persons made aware of a life threatening pre-cancerous condition would have great concern and would take immediate action. A curious phenomenon about this new form of community cancer is that while most persons agree on the diagnosis and certain spread, they choose to ignore dealing with it. We remain deaf to the growing volume of the blaring warning sirens. When we are faced with a situation for which there appears no cure, we are prone to experience a hopeless/helpless attitude that shuts down our energy factory; this has been called *psychological numbing*. Urgency demands that we wake up. Absent cure for destructive aggression of nuclear proportion, prevention stands out as our great hope.

> *The release of atomic energy has not created a new problem. It has merely*
> *made more urgent the necessity of solving an existing one.*   *... Einstein*

A Newer Way of Thinking (ANWOT) explains why our prevalent way of thinking sustains destructive aggression and the wars that have defined our history and will continue to do so. More important, it provides the now available steps we must take if we choose to answer our most universal prayers – peace of mind and world peace. The newer way of thinking we require is easy to teach and learn. Given our newest means of mass media, we can rapidly spread ANWOT at very little cost. The bigger problem is challenging our habitual way of thinking. Letting go of our established manner of thinking requires willingness to risk what has worked up to now. We must teach ourselves to think with reason and wisdom more than instinct and habit. The self-endorsement skills provided in The Short Course prepare us for the newer way of thinking and to become our own genie. As we free ourselves from instinct and habit, we empower our genie to acquire and act with wisdom for the greater good.

A Newer Way of Thinking offers three innovations that make it unique to our current self-help literature. **The first innovation** is the Seven *Word- switches* or *trigger words* that update our thinking for maturity. They are easily substituted for the common words we each learn during our early years that keep us bound to what fate and circumstance make of us. A word-switch redirects our prevalent manner of thinking to the preferred newer manner of processing data. Like a train-track switch or light switch, a single change may dramatically alter the course and outcome of action. Nature (through genes) and our nurturers program word meanings into every native language that bias the way we think. Thinking guided by instinct and habit is the prime source of both personal and global conflict, prejudice, and bigotry.   This is the reason we define our history by our wars. These simple word substitutions redirect the manner we process data from *instinct* and *habit* to *reason* and *wisdom*, the basis for cooperation, love, and peace. We will sustain destructive aggression as long as our thinking is dominated by nature's *fight or flight* instinct and our nurture's prevalent culture which imbeds *either ... or* (right/wrong, good/bad, us/them, for/against, mine/yours) thinking into every language.

The second innovation is The Mental Response Control Panel. It equips our will to recognize and consistently apply the "magical" Problem-solving sentence that consistently directs us to wise action and the Self-endorsement mental response pattern that is the key to patience and creating concern for the well-being of others. The regular application of these means of processing information replaces the more common harmful response patterns such as the Blaming Response that accounts for most destructive aggression, the Helpless/Hopeless "give up" pattern that shuts down our energy factory, and the Worry pattern leading to inappropriate anxiety. The Seven Word Substitutions and The Mental Response Control Panel that create a newer way of thinking are easy to teach and learn because they are clearly defined.

The third potent innovation in <u>A Newer Way of Thinking</u> is Life's Wisdom, my lifelong collection of the mental skills that others have demonstrated contribute to a successful life experience. We recognize many individuals who are endowed with the material benefits most seek – wealth, status, good looks, fame, being "right" and God's favorite, and so on who are nevertheless quite miserable; while some, absent silver spoons, even lacking in physical health, manage to create a joyous life. Life's Wisdoms are the specific mental skills we learn from those who "make it" in spite of what fate and circumstance bring. These wisdoms are also easy to teach and to learn. As it is said, we benefit by standing on the shoulders of those giants who precede and teach us.

The Seven Word-switches, the Mental Response Control Panel, and Life's Wisdoms comprise the self-teaching curriculum that frees our will from its early masters and empower us to make our own prayers a reality. I regard the mental skills leading to ANWOT as seeds requiring nourishment. My hope is to inspire you and others to become an *"each one, teach one"* who will make ANWOT as standard in our education as the ABC's. The payoff from a newer way of thinking promises to be huge because when a necessary ingredient is missing, the addition of even a small amount will be dramatic, as evidenced when a tiny dose of thyroid hormone or vitamin B[12] is added where there is a lack. Our society has yet to offer the skills Einstein foresaw that we require to survive and thrive in our Nuclear Age. We need to create the resources in our educational institutions that teach us how to live in addition to teaching us to make a living. I am convinced Einstein's insight that our short and long-term survival requires a newer way of thinking is correct. This is why I invest my energy to arouse your philanthropic interests to join me in making a newer way of thinking a common reality.

<u>A Newer Way of Thinking</u> differs from other *self*-help books because in addition to peace of mind it explains what we must do if we choose to attain peace in the world, to survive <u>and</u> thrive. It provides the skills for *doing good* as well as *feeling good*. I have combined my training in psychiatry with my peacenik interests to propose the newer way

of thinking we require to prevent Armageddon. You will learn the incredulously simple *thought control* skills that free our will from the prejudices of instinct and habit. They provide us the mental freedom to become our own person and best friend. Let's educate our thinking to consistently work <u>for</u> us and become our most potent weapon for mass construction!

The recent explosive creation of knowledge has thrust us into a new era.* Weapons of mass destruction have changed nature's long established "survival of the fittest" rule to "destruction of the fittest" because we know the fittest are the first targeted. Unlike bullets that target one individual, a single hydrogen weapon targets populations and cities; multiple bombs target civilization! If there is an aftermath, we then face polluted water and air and the consequences of damaged genes.

***The rapidity of change in this New Era* of Human Selection may be summarized as follows:**

APPROXIMATE TIMELINE OF YEARS TO → → → →	PRESENT:
EARTH → → → → → → → → → → → → →	4,600,000,000
BIOLOGIC LIFE, NATURAL SELECTION, SURVIVAL OF THE FITTEST → → → → → →	3,800,000,000
EXTINCTION OF DINOSAURS → → → → → → → → → → →	65,000,000
HOMO SAPIENS - AN ENLARGED BRAIN → → → → → → → → →	2,000,000
HUMANKIND ---BEGINNING OF CIVILIZATION, **AND PREVALENT MANNER OF THINKING** → → →	500,000
REFINEMENT OF LANGUAGE: HUMAN SELECTION JOINS NATURAL SELECTION → → → →	50,000
EVIDENCE OF ART AND CREATIVITY → → → → → → → → → →	30,000
MASS MEDIA & COMMUNICATION, COMPUTERS, AND FAST "EVERYTHING": TRAVEL/FOOD/ETC. → →	100
NEW ERA: WMD/WMC, **DESTRUCTION OF THE FITTEST**, HUMAN SELECTION TRUMPS NATURAL SELECTION →	60
?? ANWOT, CONSTRUCTIVE AGGRESSION, WMC/~~WMD~~ → → → → → → → → → → →	??
WMC = weapons of mass construction; WMD = weapons of mass destruction	

Modern science is providing us knowledge of our Neanderthal ancestors some 40,000 – 50,000 years past. We may assume that the road to civilization began about then. Imagine life before cultivation of food, when sustenance depended on wandering from place to place in search for plants and what one could kill. There were no permanent residences and virtually nothing material to own but primitive weapons, women, and children. Writing would not be invented for another 10,000 years, and primitive art and written accounts of history would require an additional 10,000 years. Being limited in language skills (no classes in reading and writing!), would you imagine what "meanings" would be prominent in their manner of thinking? How would civilization be passed on from generation to generation? How far have we come? How far do we have to go?

We have discovered the link between apes and humans; it is us! *Humane* includes the qualities of kindness, mercy, compassion, and concern for the welfare of humankind. We aren't there yet. We're still part animal, part human. At issue is how much of each? We must educate ourselves in ANWOT if we choose to make ourselves more humane. It took us a long time to accept that we are not the center of our universe. Those brave enough to suggest it did not have an easy time. The establishment more than resisted.

We got over it. We are keenly aware that every quantum leap innovation that challenges established thinking will meet resistance, as prominently demonstrated by Christ, Copernicus, Galileo, Columbus, Darwin, Einstein, Freud, Gandhi, Martin Luther King, Picasso, Fawcett/Pankhurst/Susan B. Anthony,[23] Al Gore, and so many others. We'd like to believe we're a step beneath the angels. If they do exist, our conception of them would require us to conclude that we are much closer to apes, an assumption for which we do have considerable scientific evidence.

Humankind is unique by its ability to think. We mentally process physical information to mental alternatives, choose among the creations we initiate, and will them to action. $E=mc^2$ explained that mass could be converted to immense energy. This knowledge led to "the bomb." Do you recognize that **the cortical portion of our brain, our organ equipped for *mental freedom*, <u>routinely</u> converts physical signals, i.e. mass, into mental energy in the form of abstract concepts and then back again to physical action?** We call this mysterious mind-body phenomenon *will power*. "Humanmind" grows, stores, and shares knowledge. The *meaning* assigned to symbols creates the energy[24] that is our source of *will* power. The manner we think determines how our will converts the mental energy of concepts into physical action.

For the first time, an earth creature has empowered its will with the godlike power to dramatically change itself <u>AND</u> the world shared by all life, a world that until this instant in time has been the sole domain of nature. *Humanmind* has joined *natural selection* in directing our destiny! We are now partner with those forces that have forever past made us what we are and determine what we may become. Our manner of thinking is no longer adequate to preserve us in this New Era. The nuclear age has instantly changed Nature's long established *survival* of the fittest rule to *destruction* of the fittest. We will remain on a course to self-destruction until we assume mastery of our will power and educate our freedom organ to become our weapon for mass <u>con</u>struction (WMC). **The technology we now have for mass education along with our collective wisdom is sufficient to thrive in our New Era. Read on to see how we may proceed to succeed; we need only create the spark that initiates our will!**

It has become popular to argue that organized religion is the cause of most of our ills, including wars, while others provide good evidence to refute this. For example, we could blame political and economic issues, conflict between the haves and the have-nots, desire for power and dominance to control others, ethnicity, skin color, jealousy, and so on.[25] Such blaming detracts us from the germane issue that **the meaning assigned to data determines the degree that thinking acts for our well-being and/or to our detriment.** The common element in harmful aggression has been and remains the manner our human mind thinks. No other creature engages in such blaming, resentment, passes hate on to future generations, creates guilt, demands recognition and a rewarded afterlife as do we.

---

[23] Leaders of the suffragette movement giving women the right to vote.

[24] Does the word "fire" trigger the same amount of energy in a language not understood by the individual?

[25] I personally believe that our most popular religions are dominated by advocates of those qualities that promote our humanity and peace. Religious leaders are among our most important force to bring about the nirvana we seek. Once aroused from passivity, they offer the best hope to reform those radical fundamentalists that would bring harm to every "other."

We may say, "I think, therefore I am dangerous."

The manner we think has been and continues to be responsible for both destructive AND constructive aggression, war and peace, prejudice and tolerance, hatred and love. Education to upgrade our thinking to meet the new challenges we face offers our best hope to attain the nirvana we seek while avoiding self-destruction along the way. The ANWOT mental skills provided here are easily taught and easily learned. The resources we require are immediately available. We need only choose to direct our will to make the effort.[26]

The most potent cause of our current ills will be found by recognizing that when we blame, our bent trigger finger points at our *self, specifically* our prevalent manner of thinking. In pointing the finger inward, we need to include our society. Establishment mores and laws are an expression of the dominant manner individuals think. Most persons remain dependent on their first masters because we have yet to institutionalize the education we require to upgrade our thinking for maturity. When we (mis)perceive that we are powerless to change "the other," and/or "the establishment," our common response is apathy, the mental equivalent of the instinctive physical *flight* pattern. Perhaps this explains the epidemic of psychological deafness to the **red alert** sirens blaring throughout the world. **With a modicum of self-endorsement skill, the seven simple word changes here to be explained are sufficient to free our thinking from domination by those early programmers of our native language and their perspectives regarding harmful aggression.**

Nature has gifted us its newest brain, the cerebral cortex that I call our "freedom organ." Our *nurturers* have provided us language. These are gifts we could not refuse. Our marvelous brain paired with sophisticated language offer us our uniqueness, mental freedom from the constraints of instinct and habit. These "parents" have equipped us to fly on our own, and they are pushing us out of the nest. *Self*-mastery frees our will to pursue the wisdom that consistently promotes those humane qualities we presently preach more so than teach. Thus far, we have used our two gifts to create science. Science expands knowledge. Power and creativity flow from knowledge. Humankind's attainment of unprecedented power and creativity is dangerous when directed by instinct and habit. These behaviors have been designed to be adaptive for animals and our own prolonged period of physical and mental immaturity. Inherent in power is a need to apply it wisely. Mental freedom empowers us to direct our life's experience for our betterment AND for our detriment. ANWOT conveys that we ourselves have the responsibility to add wisdom to our growing mental freedom. We increasingly decide to what degree we direct our aggressive energy to constructive and/or destructive outcomes. Our life's experience and of those we create are now literally in our own "head." Adding wisdom to power is an active choice available to a freed will. A **freed will + wisdom** is our formula to choose peace, to become our own genie and make our wishes a reality. Given a choice, favoring the development of wisdom or the creation of physical power, we can understand that thinking dominated by instinct would initially make physical might a clear priority. Though we invest in both, consider how heavily we invest in physical weapons

---

[26] "*Good Aggression*" in chapter 4 explains in great detail *why* and *how* we may succeed.

of destruction and defense. Let's upgrade our thinking to recognize that the power of wisdom provides greater security and permanence than physical might.

WHY A NEWER WAY OF THINKING?
You are needed

<u>A Newer Way of Thinking</u>, ANWOT is a collection of the mental skills we require if we choose to free our will from what nature and our nurturer's prejudices have made of us. This process of attaining mental freedom has also been called *becoming our own person* and *self*-mastery. We are our own enemy because destructive aggression is inherent in the manner we think. We have become our worst enemy because we have recently become so powerful that we create weapons of mass destruction for which there is no cure. We are recklessly changing the world so that it will no longer be able to provide our needs.

Einstein recognized that our prevalent manner of thinking is the root cause of our contemporary problems and is no longer adequate to protect us from our *self*. As one author put it, "We are doing better and feeling worse."[27]   Though we have become our worst enemy, we also have the potential to become our own best friend. The ANWOT skills are so simple to learn that most will be incredulous that they so powerfully advance us along the road to humanity and civilization. The ANWOT mental skills will make a huge difference because there is such a deficiency in these *mental vitamins*. Our established educational system has yet to make ANWOT education standard in its curricula.

Knowledge is our resource for both shared prosperity and global disaster, or some combination of them. Our recent explosion of scientific knowledge has thrust us into a New Era where *human selection* is replacing *natural selection*. After WWII, sufficient nuclear bombs were stockpiled to destroy the world as we know it 100 times over. Cure may no longer be within our options. The only defense where cure is unlikely is prevention. We must popularize ANWOT if we are to thrive and survive the threats of modernity. Einstein not only ushered in this New Era where *human selection* is joining *natural selection* in determining our fate; he also told us what we must do to prevent Armageddon. The tick-tick-ticking of the doomsday clock is approaching midnight. Einstein's prophecy is correct … it is only a matter of time until we create our own "big bang." Each of us is a member of a larger system that is on a course to destruct. Someone(s) will unleash destructive power never before experienced and unimaginable by most persons.

To illustrate the need for a newer way of thinking, join me on a brief visit to a fantasized planet, one that has some similarities to our own. Would you imagine a planet with seven distinct continents, each containing among its creatures a family of humanoids (the H's). On each continent, there is struggle for dominance. Through their smarts, the H's come to dominate all other creatures. The H's on each continent develop their own culture, customs, beliefs, and rules that actually increase their dominance. Though the cultures on each continent differ, they each live harmoniously within their confines, unaware that there are other continents with a distinct system of life and assumptive views. Each population is obedient to, even fiercely protective of, their own set of beliefs and rules. As the families

---

[27]   *Doing Better and Feeling Worse*, John H. Knowles (Ed.), Norton and Company, Inc., N.Y. 1977.

on each continent grow more knowledge, they improve their means of communication and travel. They discover the world extends beyond their continent; they are no longer isolated from one another. Indeed, their growing means of travel and communication "shrinks" their world. H's now confront other H's who appear unfamiliar, speak a different tongue, and fail to obey the rules of their established cultures. What would you predict of the confrontation of H's of these different continents? Thus far, each family has confronted other creatures that they have dominated through superior power. It has been quite acceptable to consider all non-H's objects suitable to service their bidding: to provide food, labor, and amusement. To make a servant and/or kill any non-H has been the law of the land. It seems quite predictable that each family of H's would first use their intelligence as they have in the past, to grow more physical power and so dominate the "other." Each family directs its energy and intelligence to produce greater power, viz. weapons of mass destruction. Their efforts result in great success. Each family of H's produces the destructive mega-power to unquestionably diminish whoever would challenge their authority.

Yet there is a problem. Einstein foresaw the problem. As founding father of our new age of mega-power, he recognized that our nature and nurture destined us to use our intelligence to include destructive means along with constructive means to attain our needs and wants. Our mastery of science enables us to make such powerful destructive weapons that we no longer preserve our lives at the expense of others. Rather, we take our own lives along with that of others. Nature's perspective, *(physical) might makes right* is no longer adequate; it is but partially true.

Do you understand his concern? As long as H's continue to think as they have been accustomed, it is merely a matter of time before Armageddon, mass mutual destruction! Perhaps more insightful than the $E=mc^2$ equation that led to *the bomb*, Einstein provided a solution to the danger he prophesied. *We shall require a substantially new manner of thinking if mankind is to survive,* one that will direct our intelligence to act with *reason* and *wisdom* more so than instinct and habit. We need to update our operating system so that it can consistently direct our mega-powers to constructive outcomes. To what avail is Nirvana if we self-destruct along the way?

As our recent science of travel and communication shrinks our world into an interrelated global economy, the "us" also grows bigger. "Me" is increasingly becoming a part of a larger "us." As the "us" grows larger in size, the number of "us's" diminishes; the trend is towards a divided world where there is only one "us" and one or a few of "them." Each is intent on domination and forcing the "other" to accept their political and/or religious assumptions. Given our historical and present perspective favoring destructive aggression and the explosive growth of our power to make a difference, it is clear we are headed for holocaust of unimaginable proportion … unless we provide new direction!

In our own not too distant past, every person was armed with two fists. Gradual weapons sophistication resulted in a few having guns, then many having them, and in some areas, most. Nobel's discovery of dynamite produced bombs (and the Nobel Peace Prize!), which have become quite commonplace. The suicide bomber is a current "innovation." Now the number of groups possessing multiple weapons of mass destruction is increasing, as are the individuals who could trigger them with the push of a button or simple utterance. Given our present manner of thinking, in which of these situations would you and your loved ones be most secure? Do you believe that increasing our physical power increases our security? I personally believe escalation of physical power may temporarily serve as a source of deterrence; it is certainly not a long-term solution to preserve our well-being.

We have created this critical time of both danger and opportunity through rational thinking. Scientific discovery is the product of the cooperation of our collective mental energy throughout our history. If two heads can be more productive than one, imagine what is to be learned through the collected wisdom of multiple insights from each segment of humanity. **Is there any culture, religious group, race, or geographic region that cannot contribute some piece to the diversity of wisdom we require?** What is remarkable in our lifetime is the abundant wisdom in our texts, the collection of ideas in our libraries, and the ability to share information via our growing efficiency in communication. The task ahead is to persuade each culture, religious group, race, and geographic region that virtue implores love more so than hate, peace more so than war, sharing more so than hoarding, cooperation more so than dominating, freedom more so than slavery. We make such truths apparent through the reasoned outcome of wisdom. More than tolerance for others, **peace requires that we understand our <u>need</u> for the wisdom "others" have to contribute.** We may grow the momentum for global peace by initially convincing and persuading ourselves of these values, by pointing an educating finger <u>inward</u> to strengthen our personal responsibility. Some would prefer slavery to death. Who would choose slavery over freedom? Freedom cannot persist without the companion of wisdom.

Now I reaffirm the most important reason to read <u>A Newer Way of Thinking</u>. You are needed to become <u>one </u>of *each one, teach one* who will help develop and popularize the ANWOT mental skills that upgrade our thinking to deal with our most universal unresolved problem … destructive aggression. ANWOT frees our will power from the prejudices of our genes and nurturers. A freed will + wisdom empower us, through our freedom organ, to act with knowledge and wisdom more than instinct and habit. We need to become the genie who can answer our own prayers, that can make our wishes a reality. Along the way we first acquire the prerequisite skill to global peace: peace of mind. If I have not yet persuaded you to become *one* to participate in ANWOT please read on.

While the benefits of ANWOT are many, consider these very important advantages of owning our thinking, of *self*-mastery, of *becoming our own person*:

1. As director and producer of our thinking, we will be free to create our own life's script including "feeling good," "doing good," and participating as a valuable member of our community.
2. We may acquire our *self* as our best friend and lifelong traveling companion. As such, we may work for and enjoy the approval of "others," by our <u>choice</u>, rather than remain a "love junkie," dependent on the whims of "others" for our well-being. We can grow our well-being independent of the weather, economics, and whoever and/or whatever we currently allow to control our react button.
3. As we create loving *self*-endorsement to fill your own needs, what overflows may be shared with others. We will experience the joy of giving.
4. We will enjoy chronic enthusiasm for the many interests <u>we</u> our *self* choose to pursue during our lifetime. By originating our own ideas and problem-solving, we will experience the "aha!" "eureka!" *self*-rewarding mental and emotional orgasms that so endear us to freedom.
5. When we ourselves are no longer servants to fate and circumstance, we become better role models to teach our children to enjoy the freedom of thought and creativity, and to surpass this generation in knowledge and achievement.[28]
6. Keep in mind that the state of our world is increasingly an expression of how we as individuals think.

You could certainly add to this list.

What <u>A</u> <u>N</u>ew <u>Way</u> <u>of</u> <u>T</u>hinking (ANWOT) can do for you

☐ Are you your own best friend or your worst enemy? You are with yourself far more than any other person. Become your own best friend and great traveling companion.

☐ Do you have difficulty expressing love? Is it easier to carry resentment? Grow your skill in love-making as you let go of resentment.

☐ Seven easy to acquire mental skills will turn your manner of thinking into your most powerful weapon for mass <u>construction</u> (WMC).

☐ Grow your patience by teaching yourself the skill of *emotional* self-endorsement.

☐ The Mental Response Control Panel will equip your will to act using the two choices that consistently work for you while avoiding the six that usually are trouble.

☐ You need not obsess wasting energy deciding which is the right decision? Teach yourself to make your decisions right!

☐ Do others control your "react button?" Some who you'd least want to? Pull it in and get your own hand on it. It's quite easy.

☐ Does anger and aggression get you into trouble? Learn to direct your energy to get you what you want and avoid what you don't want.

☐ Are you still haunted by the "shoulds" that others have programmed into you? Free yourself to be your own person.

[28] An insight of Thurayya al-Urayyid: "There is no hope of continued survival for a nation that deprives it youngsters of the ability to think and to add to the growth of human progress." *Hartford Courant*, 5/12/03, A-11.

☐ Do you still understand the world in the *either...or*, good <u>or</u> bad, right <u>or</u> wrong manner you were taught? Learn to open your mind; get a better grip on reality.

☐ Most important, acquire the basic skills to feel good and do good.

☐ Free your creative energy to work in the best interest of your *self*.

☐ Recognize that you *have* the five ingredients you need to take charge of your life.

☐ Are you preoccupied with your "worry pedestal"? Why not trade it in for an "optimism pedestal"?

☐ Do you let anxiety keep you from living your life? Challenge the "what ifs" that imprison you and overcome your fears.

☐ You can make this book your most important read, certainly within the top five!

☐ **Would you like to become a potent source for peace in the world? <u>A Newer Way of Thinking</u> explains how you may inspire others to contribute to the solution rather than remain part of the problem. Experience chronic enthusiasm as you make yourself an important member of the greater system to which you are a part.**

Let's understand that *self*-mastery is more than being creative and doing good. *Self*-mastery is the unprecedented power to change the direction of fate's prescribed course, to plot one of our own design, to take a leadership role in our own personal destiny. If our genes and nurturers have prescribed a very good set of directions for us to get along in the world, we may already have a wonderful life experience. We may be creative; we may receive praise for our good works. But our life's direction is still at the behest of some other's will. If we apply the directions provided in the ANWOT's practical strens, they will likely further increase our satisfaction. However fulfilling, as long as we remain the "muscle" following the directions provided by some "other," we have not truly attained *self*-mastery. We will be following a course like an arrow shot out of a bow. The ANWOT <u>Guide</u> will simply be another "archer" added to the long line of nurturers who have determined our life's course. The mental skills are not meant to simply add to the list of directions to our thinking. The desired outcomes are (1) that we transform "directions" from our genes and nurturers into information and knowledge for our consideration, (2) that we use our power of reflective thinking to wisely validate ("valudate") the perspectives we have passively received from "others," and (3) independently confirm and/or originate our <u>own</u> assumptions, beliefs, and values supported by reason and wisdom more so than instinct and blind obedience.

The wonderful news is that we now have both the knowledge and resources to make our mind our weapon for mass construction. <u>A Newer Way of Thinking</u> explains why we are part of the problem and how each of us can become an important force to spread peace in the world. The same technology that has enabled us to create weapons of mass destruction (WMD) is available to direct our energy for peace of mind and peace in the world. ANWOT is now quite doable. Mass communication makes it possible to share our accumulated and collective knowledge ... to rapidly educate our masses ... at little or no cost ... at our own preferred location and time.

You will learn why historically and presently, prejudice, intolerance, hatred, war, and destructive aggression are rooted in every native language. Our prevalent manner of thinking is the source of blame, "guilt," worry, resentment, depression and the ills that detract from our quality of life. Love (perhaps our most potent force), happiness, concern, forgiveness, cooperation, philanthropy, sharing, and the direction of our mental energy to create *weapons of mass construction* (WMC) are also expressions of the manner we think. Each of us is dominated by a similar manner of thinking, no matter how our race, color and/or geographic location differ. Our early manner of thinking is initially programmed by two powerful masters, our *genes* and our *nurturers* to serve their perspectives. Both advocate destructive aggression! We inherit the survival of the fittest "fight or flight" instinct to obtain our *needs*. Our prevalent culture teaches us symbolic means to dominate others to obtain our *wants* … through political, economic, and religious means. Wars will persist until we popularize ANWOT. The Newer Way of Thinking provides those mental skills that empower us to make a difference: becoming our own best friend, freeing our thinking from those prejudged demands that no longer work, and identifying the wisdom(s) that empowers us to make our collective will power our WMC. Please help make our world a kinder, gentler place for ourselves, those we love, and all of our neighbors.

Let's consider what most people want: life, power, wealth, and freedom. People today tend to strive for physical wealth more than *mental* wealth. They seek money, gold, jewels, toys for children, and special "adult toys" for grown-ups. What toys would you like to own? What is your idea of power and wealth? If a genie were to grant you several wishes, would you include the wish for mental wealth?

Most persons want to be rich not only for themselves, but also desire to enrich their loved ones. This is why we make a will – instructions of what we want to happen to our material goods when we are no longer here to enjoy them. My most memorable trip was to New Guinea. There, among other things, I learned what it took to become most respected - "a Big Man." Power and wealth were not enough; to become a Big Man, one must share his wealth with members of the tribe. Since one's ownership of pigs was the primary measure of wealth, the Big Man regularly provided feasts for all to enjoy. The "Big Man politician" became powerful according to the amount of benefits he obtained for the tribe from the central ruling body.

In your lifetime have you received something of value from some other(s) that was freely given, that actually provided satisfaction to the giver? Perhaps you have thought of what you might want to bequeath to your loved ones. Most people do not acquire a great deal of material wealth. Have you ever considered gifting your **mental** wealth to those you love? Few have, few formally do so! **Mental wealth is wisdom we attain through the mental muscles we call "thinking."** Mental wealth includes, among other assets, the skills that create *self*-worth (the minimum daily requirement of self-endorsement), meaning, companionship (especially being a good friend to one's *self*), peace of mind, happiness, enthusiasm, health, and the many mental tools that build well-being. We may increase our mental wealth throughout our lifetime. Every person with even a modest amount of intelligence can acquire and own mental wealth. And one does not have to wait to die to give it away. The curious thing about giving away your mental wealth is that the more you give, the more you acquire. And if you document your mental wealth (there are many ways to do so), you can create a substantial inheritance for those you love. Consider documenting the most meaningful lessons you learn in your lifetime on a tape or computer disk to bequeath to your loved ones. Would you cherish such a gift from the important people in your life who have passed on?

Our physical and mental muscles are our basic sources of power and freedom. Mental strength is relatively easy to grow and considerably easier to pass on to others than physical strength. Our physical muscles consist of many strands. With exercise, they increase in size and strength. Working together, they provide us the physical strength to exercise our will. If you were a slave, your muscles would serve to exercise someone else's will. How we abhor being someone else's slave. Mental muscles, like physical muscles, also consist of many strands. Each strand contributes to our collective wisdom. Wisdom is our most basic resource to get us what we want; it is stronger and has more endurance than our physical muscles. Single strands of wisdom are most effective when bunched together, as are our physical muscles. While we inherit our physical muscles, the strands of mental muscles that provide us will power and freedom need be acquired. Like the physical muscles that free our body, the wisdom to free our mind also requires exercise. I label each strand of mental strength a "stren." Collect strens, exercise them, and you will grow mentally strong. The mental wealth we acquire is limited primarily by our willingness to work and exercise our strens. Most persons regularly exercise their physical muscles; few have a routine to grow our mental muscles.

It is said our wisdom is largely the result of the opportunity we have to stand on the shoulders of the giants who have preceded us. A Newer Way of Thinking (ANWOT) is an exercise program of the wisdom of such giants, presented in bits-and-pieces, as strens. Each strand, or stren, will add the mental muscle that empowers us to get what we need, what we want. ANWOT is the growing collection of the strens I have obtained from others (most, willingly offered) and share with you. Their wisdom is presented in a format that can be easily understood, acquired, customized to one's personal life situation, expanded, and passed on to others. I hope you will accept them from my free offering, "steal" them[29], modify them, add to them, and/or create new ones, identify them as your own, apply their wisdom, and perhaps, even give back some in new or better condition than the ones I offer.

The urgency to prevent the unleashing of our WMD has never been greater. Within my generation, we have created and spread such unprecedented destructive power that recovery from its negative consequences may no longer be assured; "cure" is rapidly becoming extinct. Wisdom demands that we create a newer way of thinking to direct our mental energy.

Here is why success is ours if we only exercise our collective will:
☼ Mental freedom from the demands of instinct and habit, nature and our nurturers, fate and circumstance, is among our most sought after goals. Skill in *thought control* emancipates our will to direct our own life's experience.
☼ ANWOT is easy to teach and learn and may readily be embraced by the masses of all cultures. Communication technology and computers make it available at little or no cost in one's own home and/or convenient location.

[29] Written permission is required if used for profit. Reference to this book will help spread ANWOT.

☼ The skills to feel good and do good are universally desired.

☼ How many are for peace of mind, peace for humankind? How many against? Strens emphasize the wisdom which, when added to *self*-mastery, directs our energy to weapons of mass construction more so than weapons of mass destruction.

☼ We far more prefer those common values universally recognized by philosophers and preached by our religions than those that stir conflict. We want to create the utopian world that is within our capability.

☼ The blaring sirens warning us of the impending use of weapons of mass destruction are increasingly difficult to ignore. They are a promising source of motivation.

MENTAL FREEDOM: THE GIFT OF *SELF*-MASTERY WE CAN REFUSE

Freedom is among our most cherished wants; some hold freedom to be even more important than life itself. Slavery is universally abhorred, certainly if one's role is slave rather than master. Most everyone reading this manual is *physically* a free person while few have attained true *mental* freedom. The Emancipation Proclamation of 1863 freed the *muscles* of slaves. Deprived of education and opportunity to free their mind, many were initially worse off than when directed by a benevolent "master". *Physical* freedom unleashes the power of muscle. *Mental* freedom is taking control of our will power from the early masters of our life's experience to direct our thinking, feelings, and actions.

Each of us, yes, you and I included, are required to serve the whims of fate and circumstance. And most of us, although convinced of our independence, remain imperceptibly a mental servant to those masters who first create our life's script. What higher goal is there than liberating our mind "to pursue our own good in our own way" (John Stuart Mill)? Imagine owning the *something* that gives us the power to consistently *feel good* and *do good*? Who likes having "others" write their life's script? Most prefer to become their own director and producer. The following examples convey why mental freedom is among the most valuable possessions we can acquire.

What is it about each person's behavior that seems *wacko, yet* I consider *normal*?
1. Jenny, ten years old, was quite happy and singing when prevented just in time from hanging herself.
2. Mike was a bully. He hated blacks and Jews and threatened to blow up his high school.
3. Susan could not sleep comfortably unless she had cotton in her mouth.
4. Joe was regularly put in the prison "hole" (isolation) for sexual attack on other young inmates.
5. Grace was convinced she was possessed by Lucifer, the devil.
6. Jacob threw up upon the thought of eating this food.
7. By the age of three, these children already hated all Catholics while a comparison group already hated all Protestants.
8. Kamikaze pilots during WWII and suicide bombers in the mid-East conflict disregard one of our most powerful instincts – survival.

They each were behaving just as they had been taught! Their feelings and actions were quite normal responses to the way their early masters had programmed their manner of thinking.

1. Jenny was told that when she died she could again be with her favorite person, her deceased grandmother.

2. Mike's mom was abandoned by the man who impregnated her. Middle class but unable to cope, she drifted lower and lower on the economic scale, was raped twice, and vented her bitterness and prejudiced opinions through her son.

3. Susan was convinced by her superstitious mom that something terrible would happen to mom if she didn't regularly chew cotton at night. Her peers laughed at her when she revealed her secret at a pajama party. It took some time and many restless nights to get use to sleeping without her cotton.

4. Joe "knew" he had to ejaculate to get rid of a "tight collar" but also that it was a sin to spill his seed outside of flesh. Once his opinion was exposed in a group therapy session, and he was persuaded by his peers that it was O.K. to "beat the meat," I no longer had to see him in the seclusion cell to determine an appropriate disciplinary action.

5. Grace was brought up where speaking in tongues and hearing voices were expected occurrences during the prayer rituals. She was admitted to my care when I was a resident in psychiatry at Johns Hopkins because she was suicidal, convinced she was evil. Her religious leader confirmed that in his opinion she was indeed possessed.

6. Jake discovered the roast beef sandwich was actually ham; he realized he violated his religion's dietary code and immediately vomited. As a college student, I witnessed a similar situation when Mohammed, having been assured there was no meat in the vegetable stew, found on his spoon what was unmistakably a piece of bacon.

7. Observed in a study of children growing up in Ireland [Hartford Courant, 7/25/02]. What might we expect of a child growing up in Palestine? In Israel? Wherever unresolved conflict is common?

8. Through years of immaturity, their way of thinking was indoctrinated by leaders who chose to keep themselves isolated from the sights, sounds, and smells of murder.

What prejudgments yet control <u>your</u> thinking? Free your will. Become your own genie.

Some compare our freedom organ to a *tabula rasa*, an unwritten-on tablet. Like a computer or robot, it is first programmed according to the whims of those who do the programming. This is why the same morsel of meat (pork or beef) that results in delightful anticipation by one individual is a source of revulsion in an individual whose cultural upbringing forbids eating it. Even simple symbols such as a cross, a crescent, a six-pointed star and/or a swastika can summon powerful but totally opposite thoughts and emotions according to one's early training. We can understand why some "leaders" who have decades to program immature minds may easily create martyrs, kamikaze pilots, and suicide bombers while they themselves characteristically isolate themselves from the sights, sounds, and smells of human destruction. How shall we explain why, throughout history, virtually every religion honors those who create harm to nonbelievers in the name of their God? Is God confused?

Throughout our first decades the way we process information is dominated by the two masters that make us what we are. These masters are identified by various labels: our genes and culture, nature and our nurturers, fate and circumstance, the potential we inherit and what our early programmers make of our thinking. **Mental freedom is the process of adding a third master, _self_-mastery, to the first controllers of our destiny. ANWOT consists of those mental skills that convey ownership of our thinking, that free our will from domination by "other" masters, that create _genie hood_.** We alone among earth's creatures have a _freedom organ_, the cortical portion of our brain. Its size and complexity is sufficient to direct and produce our life's experience through the discipline of developing our mental muscles – _will power_ and _wisdom_. Through our accumulated knowledge -- our rapidly expanding sciences -- human selection is now joining natural selection to determine our fate. _Humanmind_, properly educated with mature thinking skills and knowledge, provides us sufficient will power to overrule much of nature's and our nurturers' control over our destiny.

We are mental interpretive becomings[30]! The way we think influences the way we feel and the way we act. The _meanings_ of words and symbols govern our manner of thinking. Meanings are first programmed by "others." ANWOT is the programming _we_ create to update our thinking for maturity. The process is accomplished by simple but critical word substitutions that I call _word-switches_ or _trigger words_. We require a very limited number of these trigger words to acquire the _thought control_ that powerfully influences our feelings and actions. By choosing to invest in <u>a</u> <u>n</u>ewer <u>way</u> <u>of</u> <u>t</u>hinking (ANWOT), we acquire ownership of our _self_.

Whereas other creatures are prone to respond reflexively to the data received, we are equipped to act on the _meaning_ our freedom organ assigns to the data. Other earth creatures follow destiny's course. We create, dwell, and actively intervene in our own mental _virtual_ world. We study the rules, challenge and modify them. Our _freedom organ_ converts physical energy into mental energy and initiates _will_ power to convert mental energy into physical action.

nerves/hormones/etc. $\rightarrow$ concepts/thinking $\rightarrow$ will power $\rightarrow$ physical action

----

<u>_Who_ or _what_ **programs the operating systems (O.S.s) that determine the manner we think?**</u>

Our programmers include nature and our nurturers (as it is with all earth creatures) and to whatever degree we choose to program our _self_. **We may join our early masters as the third programmer of the manner we think.** Through our early years, nature and our nurturers equip the cortical portion of our brain with words and symbols that convey meaning. Our native language expresses the perspectives of our first masters and remains faithful to the meaning of the symbols they provide. Our mind uncritically accepts the meanings we are provided to process information to action. Thus, our mind's first operating systems (O.S.s) are the expression of what fate and circumstance make

---

[30] "becomings" is more accurate than "beings" because unlike other earth creatures, our freedom organ empowers us to customize who and what we become. As we acquire knowledge, store it, share it, and pass it on through generations, we grow the power of our will to change ourselves and the world. Through science, we are rapidly increasing our role as directors of our destiny, and I am told more scientists are alive today than all of history. Here is a good example of the manner our language distorts our perception of reality. "Beings" conveys we are static. Such _meaning_ constrains our creative thinking if it does not convey our opportunity for _self_-mastery. Until we equip our freedom organ with ANWOT, I suppose we are more _human beings_ than _human becomings_. [Aha - my spell checker is _on_ to indicate _becomings_ is not in our dictionary] ANWOT equips our freedom organ to function as a _human becoming_.

of us. "The gift we cannot refuse" aptly describes the dependency manner of thinking first embedded in our native language. Our early thinking has been designed to work effectively through the years that we are physically undeveloped and mentally immature. We can understand why the early O.S.s that emphasize instinct and obedience to authority are insufficient to manage the issues of our contemporary world.

Consider the world from the perspective of a child. It is a simple place where there are good guys _or_ bad guys, right _or_ wrong, rewards _or_ punishment, good _or_ evil. The meanings our genes and nurturers wire into our immature brain are passively received. Their perspective of how we are to interpret the world is etched into our early O.S.s through repetition and tempered through habit. Nurturers are required and thereby become expected to provide necessary help and care. When the world doesn't comply with our unrealistic expectations, we experience frustration and are prone to find someone or something to blame (and punish). Demands and/or a temper tantrum are in order. Such tantrums may persist into adulthood when the world is "unfair" and fails to meet our expectations. Most of us also learn the relatively unique-among-earth-creatures pattern of self-blame, i.e. guilt.

The early manner of processing information suits our helpless, dependent, nurtured state when our brain is ill-equipped and we have little sense of "_self._" Unrealistic expectations become our main source of problems to the degree we continue to use these O.S.s when we attain physical maturity. You get the idea! Our mind first functions more like an intelligent slave. It may be brilliant and creative though it yet remains servant to its first masters.

What instinct first makes of us is thereafter determined by parents and nurturers. Our _nurturers_ modify our gene's programming with meaning suitable to _their_ wants, to blindly obey _their_ authority. They provide words, _their_ meanings and values, and establish how we habitually use them. Our native language, identity, name, rules of conduct, interpretation of the world, beliefs, values, our religion, and so on are "their orders" routinely appearing in our thoughts and thinking. In our partially civilized world, the _symbols_ of power are preferred to instinct's proneness towards physical aggression. We are taught to get our wants through titles, position, wealth, owning, status, "rightness," winning in competition ("beating" others), asserting God and/or the prevalent authorities are on our side, etc. However, when symbolic dominance fails, physical aggression is condoned. The more primitive means of fighting, killing, and war may then be sanctioned. Immature thinking limits its conclusions to two categories such as right _or_ wrong, good _or_ bad, and "I (we) know what is right." This manner of thinking seeks punishment for noncompliance. Thus, the programming imbedded in our native language supports fate and circumstance's prejudged values including prejudice, hatred, intolerance, blaming others, _guilting_ our _self_, and related means that support harmful aggression.

Do you agree that **genes and our culture** are formidable "masters" of our life's experience? These "others" who first program and direct our thoughts aspire to continue as rulers of our thinking. The meanings we passively acquire express our period of blind obedience. Only the creation of a newer manner of thinking can free our will power from slavery to its early masters. Emancipation requires that we actively rewire our _meaning-_

pathways, which through years of repetition have become relatively effortless through habit.

Unlike nature's endowment of automatic <u>physical</u> maturity, we receive no program that turns on mature thinking! Rather, nature provides us "hardware," its latest, most advanced brain with the mental capacity that when mature dwarfs any computer we create. It also provides us a beginning software program we call *instinct*. Thereafter, our nurturers provide us our native language operating system (O.S.), humankind's product 50,000 years in the making. The mating of our marvelous hardware to the sophisticated language and knowledge provided by our nurturers gives birth to our unique power of *reflective thinking*. **Reflective thinking** is the capacity of our complex brain to think about our thinking, to be conscious of our consciousness. **Reflective thinking** is our resource to manipulate ideas, create and initiate new patterns, and most important to free our will from the directions of our early programmers. Do you see, we are gifted the <u>potential</u> for *self*-mastery! Mental capacity, sophisticated language, and knowledge are tools we are given to create mental freedom. **MENTAL FREEDOM IS A GIFT OF OPPORTUNITY THAT WE <u>CAN</u> REFUSE! MOST DO!**

A Newer Manner of Thinking **is the rewiring that equips our native language to deal with maturity and the challenges of modernity.** *Self*-mastery is the freedom to express our will with reason and wisdom rather than instinct and/or habit. ANWOT allows us to accept personal <u>responsibility</u> for problem-solving more so than prolonged dependency and blaming, and favors prevention over cure. I urge you to regularly apply the three critical word substitutions that free our will from "other" control:

1. *I allow* **is substituted for** *He (she, it, they) makes me.* Upgrade blaming to personal responsibility.
2. *I could* **is substituted for** *I should.* Upgrade blind obedience to rational problem-solving.
3. *Both...and* **is substituted for** *Either...or.* Upgrade thinking that forces our perception into two distorted extreme good <u>or</u> bad categories (the root of prejudice and destructive aggression) to the more accurate perception of reality that recognizes good <u>and</u> bad, the +'s <u>and</u> –'s in each of alternative choices (the basis of processing of data to constructive outcomes).

These word substitutions that I call ANWOT *word-switches* or *trigger words* redirect the dependency manner of thinking embedded in all native languages to assume *self*-mastery. The consistent use of a limited number of such substitutions powerfully upgrades our mental operating system. The fact that you are reading this guide indicates your mind is sufficiently matured and educated to acquire the skills of ANWOT. **Mental freedom is attained by educating our mind in seven simple ANWOT language upgrades to our native language O.S. Thereafter,** *The Mental Response Control Panel* **explains the eight action choices available to a freed will and identifies those two that bias our will power to consistently act with wisdom.** They are sufficient to redirect our thinking for personal responsibility, independence, choice-making among alternatives, and those qualities of mental freedom that create *self*-mastery.

Our society has yet to establish and promote the educational resources needed to bring the newer way of thinking to our masses. Our formal schooling emphasizes the three R's and the rules of our culture, the sacred perspectives etched in the "establishment." Formal education for most ceases just about the time we reach our peak receptivity to the ANWOT mental skills, when our brain has reached physical maturity, has acquired skill in the use of symbols, and is ready to learn to wisely transform knowledge into action. Multiple studies of adult development indicate that most persons aren't prepared to take control of their thinking until their late 20's, and for many, mental freedom from what our genes and nurturers make of us is never acquired. Adult educational resources are available for most any skill. Do you know of any courses in mature thinking? Our country has many institutions that teach warfare, such as the Army, Navy, Marine, and Air Force Academies, multiple colleges that are military institutes, and one scarcely funded, "shunned," virtually anonymous Peace Academy. We emphasize how to make a living while we neglect how to live. Even our "liberating" arts colleges have not targeted the skills of ANWOT for specific courses within their curriculum. How many teaching resources can you name that specialize in mental freedom and/or peace, the prizes of ANWOT? Absent such education in our primary schools and lacking adult teaching resources, we are prone to remain stuck with our early prejudices, indoctrination, and distorted thinking. The payoff will be huge because our society has so neglected education in the skills of mature thinking. Popularizing the newer way of thinking promises a quantum leap for our partially civilized world. I encourage you to become a part of the ANWOT peace academy.

ANWOT education favors *self*-mastery and mental skill-building more so than obedience to authority and inappropriate expectations that often lead to frustration, blaming, and harmful aggression. Although the percentage of persons throughout the world who have upgraded their native language for maturity and civility are small, even a small percentage of billions represents a large number of individuals. I and likely you are among the gifted minority. My nurturers have provided me a liberating education and the opportunity to be exposed to marvelous role models and teachers. If you also have been so fortunate, let me boldly suggest that you now have an obligation to do for others what has been done for you. Sharing with others what we can afford to give is an expression of becoming humane. However, here is a practical self-serving reason to spread ANWOT education to those less fortunate. To the degree we ignore the prevalent manner of thinking, of blaming leading to harmful aggression, we create and/or passively support those bigoted leaders who are the greatest threat to our well-being.

The ANWOT Curriculum educates our freedom organ for choice-making among alternatives of our own creation. It provides the following self-mastery skills:

Chapter 1 reviews the **self-endorsement skills** that enable us to become our own best friend, the required first step to freeing our thinking from domination by its early masters, instinct and habit. Masters usually resist releasing their slaves. Self-endorsement enables us to sustain the will power and risk-taking required to challenge our established manner of thinking. It enables us to personally provide the immediate reward we require when the most important benefits of our efforts come later. Self-endorsement is also our source of patience. And the excess of love we create for ourself allows us to freely and unconditionally do for others rather than *give to get*.

Chapter 2 explains our gift of the <u>opportunity</u> to acquire mental freedom. It then provides two original mental skills that enable us to challenge the prejudices of our genes and nurturers, the *prejudgments* inscribed in our thinking through *instinct* and *habit*. These two skills empower us to express our will power favoring *reason* and *wisdom*. They reprogram the manner we think to assume personal responsibility as they replace the characteristic patterns of immaturity embodied in all native languages -- dependency, blind obedience, and blaming.

    a. *Seven basic "word-switches,"* word substitutions, lead to thought control. They promote *becoming our own person* as they free our will from the dictatorship of our early programmers.

    b. *The Mental Response Control Panel* identifies the eight alternative choices available to our freed will as it transforms mental energy into physical action. Two of the choices consistently lead to beneficial outcomes while the others usually bring about what we don't want.

Simple application of three of the fully explained word-switches and consistent use of the constructive means of directing our mental energy are sufficient to create dramatic change.

Chapter 3 *is the Wisdom Collection* that others have shown guides our freed will to the constructive outcomes we desire. Power lacking wisdom is a liability more than an asset.

    Learning the ANWOT skills of self-endorsement, mental freedom, and the wisdom we require constitute the easy task. The more difficult issue is overcoming the resistance to letting-go of our established habitual manner of thinking. For those whose early teaching emphasized guilt and self-putdowns, continued practice of the mental skills of self-endorsement provided in Chapter 1 and The Short Course to Mental Wealth are especially important.

Chapter 4 explains *why* and *how* **ANWOT works**. The comprehensive essay "Good Aggression" is essential for those desiring to creatively apply ANWOT as architect and/or engineer more than as technician.

The **Glossary** defines the meanings of words and symbols conducive to a better understanding of ANWOT. **Values** that are commonly professed by our great religions, philosophers, and wise persons from our diverse culture are identified in various sections of the curriculum.

    A common science fiction theme depicts that the increasingly sophisticated robots we now create will become so smart that they will eventually "take over." They will program themselves, act independently, and seek to rule the world. Realize that <u>we are "the robot</u>," hitherto controlled by instinct and habit. We are now reprogramming ourselves to break free from the demands and commands of nature's and our nurturers' directions. By combining knowledge with skill in processing data (reflective thinking) we have become so ably *self*-programmable that we challenge our early masters. We guide our life's experience by manipulating the symbols we create and the meanings we assign to them. The *will* of *self*-mastery is becoming so powerful that it is freeing itself from the programs of our creators and early masters. In becoming the producer and director of mental action, we also empower ourselves to change the world we all share. A free *self* is capable of overruling the traditional directions we receive from the dominant controllers of our mind, *nature* through instinct, and our *nurturers* through habit.

The development of a scientific understanding of our mental trigger-power, here initiated, is the basis for acquiring *the newer way of thinking* operating system. Let us grow our freedom from fate and circumstance. Join me in empowering ourselves with <u>constructive</u> aggression to <u>wisely</u> pursue the wants <u>we</u> choose!

I have indicated that the manner we express aggression has become the most pressing unresolved threat to our survival. This is largely due to our abrupt entrance into the nuclear age and our rapid advances in technology. Though we share similarities with other earth life, **we stand apart by the degree we rely on the meanings that are assigned to symbols, our advanced second signaling system.** Meanings influence the manner we think.

Nature (genes) is first to program meanings into the symbols of our native language. The meanings nature programs into symbols stress its *fight or flight* and *survival of the fittest* perspective. Instinct biases our thinking to seek immediate satisfaction irrespective of the consequences to "the other." Our nurturers' symbols are biased to be adaptive to our decades of immaturity, before we can become our own person. Their symbols reflect our helplessness and dependency, blind obedience to authority, and need for their prejudgments regarding friend/foe, safe/dangerous, yes/no, good/bad, right/wrong, us/them, like/dislike, etc. Processing data into two categories is called *dichotomous thinking*. Such "either/or" thinking is the source of most prejudice, bigotry, hatred, destructive aggression, and ultimately war. Our inherited instinct and the meanings that we acquire from our nurturers are often contradictory.

Nature's motto is "Yes! If it feels good, looks good, and/or tastes good, and you can get away with it; do it."
Nurture's motto is "No! If it feels good, looks good, or tastes good, it's probably bad for you; don't do it ."
Each is clearly incompatible with the requirements to thrive in the new nuclear age. We may significantly enlighten ourselves by understanding how we stand apart from other life on earth.

Let's consider important attributes of four canine families: the Spaniel family, the Shepherd family, the Beagle family, and the Doberman family. Each individual and each family differs from every other. Yet, if we were to have 1000 pictures of individual family members over 15 generations, we could quite effectively sort each one into their family of origin. Our genes stress commonality amidst the great diversity between individuals. Each individual has the same predictable number of legs, and one head. Internally, each has similar organs and chemical composition. They share a like means of function. The heart pumps blood, the kidneys filter it, and bioelectrical wiring activates muscles. Each has a similar "strip" of their brain that controls voluntary muscle movement – this area is arranged in a specific fashion with the "foot movement" part on the top gradually moving to the "head movement" part, which is on the bottom. The same upside down representation of this muscle movement center in the human brain has been called a homunculus or "little person." Each member of every family has such a representation in the corresponding portion of their brain.

I find it very enlightening that each individual also has a similar specific area of the brain that deals with sexual expression, and **this same "sex" area of the brain also deals with what we call "aggressive" behavior.** Nature's way makes sense. If creatures have an interest in sexual reproductive activity but lack the aggressive urge to secure a mate, there would be no family; that family would not persist. Darwin and others have shown us that we inherit behaviors designed to maintain **the life cycle:**

birth → survive → mature → reproduce → die.

Survival requires aggressive use of our energy. Thus, **all members of the four families become quite energetic and engage in harmful <u>physical</u> aggression to preserve their life cycle. Aggressive action is of very short duration for a specific common purpose – survival from predators, obtaining food to survive, mating, and protection of the young.** Perhaps the most powerful inherited behavioral pattern in each of the above individuals is physically fighting or running to survive, the "fight or flight" instinct. Aggression is usually directed to only one at a time using basic means such as biting, clawing, making noises or gestures. Most creatures engage in destructive aggression to fulfill the life cycle, <u>not</u> for the sport of killing or destroying.

The White family from Europe, the Black family from Africa, the Red family from America, and the Yellow family from Asia, like the four-legged canine families, have a great deal in common. We predictably have two legs instead of four but have added two arms. Our organs rely on similar chemicals and electrical wiring. Yet, we significantly stand apart from all other earth creatures by the degree our conduct is guided by mental activity, specifically by the meanings we assign to words and symbols. We create an elaborate personal mental <u>second</u> world where we dwell as our primary residence. Our preferred method of experiencing life is conscious awareness and thinking using nonphysical concepts to represent physical reality. Our personal conscious awareness coexists with the common physical world we all share.[31] Through language, we have additional new means to resolve our needs beyond what we share in common with other creatures. By emphasizing words and concepts as our dominant means to process information, we also create new methods to express aggression.

Our elaborate mental function manages anger and aggression strikingly different than other earth beings. Our aggression is driven (1) by "means" more so than genes and (2) by "creed" more so than need.

(1) Our aggression is driven by "means" more so than by genes. With the development and refinement of language over the last 50,000 years, we have become increasingly dependent on "means" to determine our life style. By using words and symbols to substitute for physical reality, and by skillful mental processing of data and storage of knowledge, we have increased our flexibility, creativity, and originality. The means of survival we devise using our mental skills are favored over the preprogrammed methods we inherit. We copy what works and pass it on in perpetuity. We stand on the shoulders

---

[31] The stren *Our Two Worlds* considers the two distinct realities we must manage during our lifetime.

of the giants who preceded us. We imitate and mimic their creativity and devise better ways to share our ever-expanding knowledge. We replicate "means" as genes replicate its patterns. We have diverged from our inherited behavioral repertoire. Consider how today's sophisticated automobile has been improved from the discovery of the wheel. So it is with virtually all other aspects of our life. For example, through our chain of shared knowledge, we improve our means to preserve our health and continue to expand our means of communication and our creative and destructive power.

We no longer favor hitting and biting. By using symbols, language, and mental processing of information, we divert physical aggression to mental aggression. We seldom follow the literal *fight or flight* script provided by nature's O.S. Our nurturer's "civilized" O.S. usually forbids physical aggression. They usually succeed in teaching us to redirect physical aggression to mental means of expression. We blame others <u>and</u> ourselves. We store the urge to hurt; we feed resentment; we commonly engage in sustained "social sabotage." Such behavior is consistent with the first language we acquire when we are yet physically and mentally immature. Our native language disposes us individually to nonphysical social aggression and punishment: dominating, blaming, "beating" our opponent, taking more than we need … often to another's detriment. Through habit, it fosters prolonged dependency, conformity, and gullibility.

We prefer our nurturer's symbolic means of expressing aggression to the physical means provided by our genes. We are rapidly exceeding genetic evolution by "mimetic" change. We learn to speak and act by mimicking/copying/imitating our nurturers … and <u>their</u> perspective. Language empowers us to create and store virtual reality, to manage information, grow knowledge, to share and improve its accuracy, and to powerfully influence our common physical reality. As will be more fully explained, using words and symbols, we create choices among alternatives not available to other creatures, including new means of constructive <u>and</u> destructive aggression.

Resorting to physical aggression, including war, is usually an admission our symbolic alternatives have failed. Nevertheless, our history consists of the repetitious documentation of such failures. With astoundingly accelerating speed, we have moved from fists, slingshots, and bows and arrows, to dynamite, nuclear explosives, and chemical and biologic means for mass destructive power.

(2) As mental interpretive beings, aggression is determined by our "creeds," more so than our needs. We make assumptions to fill-in our lack of knowledge, and guide our actions by our private mental interpretations. Within our mind, our unique personal nonphysical world, we establish conscious awareness as our primary residence. Herein we participate in ongoing drama; our mind becomes the "capital" of our universe where most interpretations, assumptions, and decisions are made. **Meaning stimulates mental activity. Thoughts and thinking establish values! Values determine priorities. Priorities determine action.**

Other creatures primarily express destructive aggression using physical means to satisfy their needs. Most of their energy focuses on <u>survival</u> of their type. Our aggression is to satisfy "wants" more so than needs. **We are no longer simply prone to short term arousal to survive, get food, reproduce, protect our young, and take care of our <u>needs</u>;**

we (mentally) create, store, and commit destructive aggression to fulfill our (symbolic) wants. In our "civilized" society, aggression is no longer simply a means of individual and family survival. We strive to own the symbols of survival – money, gold, jewels, "titles" to dominate others, winning where "others" must lose, appearance, youth, owning "stuff," "God" status, being right, and -- you get the idea. We fight for freedom, status, ideology ("in the name of God"), for "principle," and when certain authorities so direct us. We seek to amass and commonly worship symbols of power and often use them to control others. "O.K." for earth's creatures is usually "enough," whereas our creed too often is "greed." *Enough* is insufficient; *more* is better. Our wants are often insatiable.

The manner we express aggression is influenced by our interpretations, beliefs, and/ or our assumptions. Our wants are commonly childlike and irrational. Individually, we demand to look a certain way, we fret over our mortality, demand that "others" provide love and sexual gratification, and anger when others are imperfect. Individually and collectively, we physically and mentally attack others simply because they belong to a different family, because they use different symbols – be it a cross, a crescent, or a star, because they have something we don't have, if they don't conduct their life the way we believe they "should," and/or don't give us what we unreasonably expect. We are also unique by the degree we commonly mentally, even physically, "attack" our self when we don't meet the usually unrealistic demands that we (and others) put to ourself.

Observation of our greater community, its customs, and its means of expressing aggression, requires the conclusion that its rules and function is a reflection of the personal manner of thinking we first learn and habitually use. This manner of thinking is becoming increasingly inefficient for our contemporary situation.

Examples of destructive aggression arising from our creeds or personal mental O.S. are ubiquitous! Simply read the newspaper: "Catholic and Protestant children start learning to fear and loathe each other's communities as young as 3 years old, a newly published study found Tuesday, blaming parents and Northern Ireland's religiously divided school system." [Hartford Courant, 7/25/02]. "Man Shoots 2 At Louisiana Airport, Says People Made Fun Of His Turban" [Hartford *Courant*, 5/23/02]. What assumptive views would you expect of a child growing up in Palestine? … or Israel? The actions of the kamikaze pilots in WWII and the suicide bombers in the mid-east conflict illustrate how "creed" overpowers physical need. Think of the many situations where culture breeds conflict more so than our nature. How commonly do you (or others) become enraged when someone breaks in line or drives too slow? Acts the way they "shouldn't?" Who/what sets off your "react button?" How do you express anger?

Rather than being disheartened and numbed by the chaos and destructive expression of our new unrestrained powers, we can envision the opportunity to create a Utopian society. We can collectively work to wisely harness the power of *self*-mastery for our benefit. Shall we welcome or disdain emancipation? Who shall we make our leader … nature, nurture, or *self*-mastery? … some combination of the three? We are the first creatures to have a choice! Reason clarifies which of our choices is wise. In this rapidly emerging new era of personal power, the directive force of instinct and habit (nature and nurture) is strong; our power for wise *self*-management is weak. While each type of "family" (white/black/red/yellow, religious, geographic, and others) preach and make rules against destructive aggression, and agree there is a better way, we have yet to develop and teach a *mental* science of thinking to consistently act according to our principles. Strens are the skills we acquire to strengthen our ability to think wisely and aggressively express constructive action. All that we need to wisely express our growing power of human selection is readily available, should we decide to provide the will.

Biologists, scientists who study living creatures, have devised a very fancy term to describe development – "Ontogeny recapitulates phylogeny." In plain language, this simply means complex creatures begin as simpler forms of life and pass through earlier patterns as they attain their most complex form. Through our individual physical conception and growth, we retrace in miniature the evolution of life.

Most earth creatures operate, from their life's start, according to the preprogrammed instinctual patterns characteristic of their nature; they are "brainless." More complex creatures are "sentient" … they are conscious of the sensations they experience. Such creatures usually have brains of varying sizes and experience a period of dependence and nurturance, the length of which corresponds to their brain size and its complexity. Habit is added to their instinctual means of operation as they acquire new patterns from outside sources after birth.   Many such creatures have conscious awareness, think, and are creative; yet, their mental skills primarily remain bound to serve the instinct and habit patterns of operation programmed by nature and their nurture. **By adding language to our mental operating system, we empower *self*-mastery with unprecedented freedom. We significantly challenge the inherited and habitual programs provided by nature and our nurturers. <u>We</u> make a difference!**

We not only influence our own destiny; we have recently jumped to a new plateau of power. We are dramatically modifying our universe. We created scientific method within a mere several hundred years. As the number of scientists and scientific discoveries grow, we are awed by both the rapidity of change and the steady *acceleration* of our ability to change. We have expanded our means of travel from foot and ass to our rapid mechanical means with the brevity of a moment in history. Compare the few generations needed to create our means for mass destruction with the period of time aggression has been limited to fists and weapons that kill one or a few at a time! The gene pool that nature provides us has been refined, in evolutionary time, over several billion years. Our ancestors required about 50,000 years to bring our sophisticated use of symbols and the mental processing of data to our contemporary state of *self*-mastery. On an <u>individual</u> personal basis, we acquire our genetic inheritance in about 9 months. We commonly take a leisurely 15-30 years to attain our individual physical and mental maturity.

How long will it take to establish an ANWOT operating system suited to wisely express the power of *self*-mastery, to direct our personal destiny, to effectively challenge the ways of nature and nurture, change our world, and perhaps even the universe? How long shall we take to develop the O.S. that is appropriate for our new godlike powers? That is readily teachable, learnable and spreadable? That adds the wisdom to consistently direct power to <u>constructive</u> outcomes? That more sharply perceives nonphysical goods and values … *feeling good* and *doing good*, love, and the joys of cooperation, sharing, and giving? Do we have an unlimited time to create this new manner of thinking? How can we proceed? We pride ourselves in mastering physical reality while we permit the mental virtual reality that is our means of control to run amuck! We invest in physical science while we virtually ignore the science of thinking. We rely on primitive obsolete methods to manage aggression. Our times demand that we teach ourselves to <u>act</u> with wisdom and not <u>react</u> from instinct and/or habit.

The physical power of *self*-mastery if directed by the mental O.S. of nature and/or nurture results in a mismatch! Consider the destructive consequences of our new powers expressed through the "survival of the fittest" O.S. of instinct and/or the mental "blaming" posture commonly acquired during the immature period of our nurturance. Soon after World War II, each major "side" had created sufficient nuclear bombs to destroy all of humanity multiple times over.[32] Now, each side focuses their resources to add newer destructive means that could achieve a similar outcome. The enormity of the power attained through physical science predisposes us to self-destruction. Power without wise direction is a liability <u>and</u> an asset. It is our nature to engage in destructive aggression. Habit has thus far resisted making way for wisdom. Indeed, the countries that have amassed the greatest knowledge have also created the most global means for destructive aggression.

The predictable harm our current path will create for "us" and "them" is compelling reason to energetically work towards wise direction of our mental power. We also observe an interesting phenomenon, the growing fear of an alien "other" that may help modify our world view into a unified cooperative "us." "They," the "others," are more commonly portrayed in our fictional media and entertainment as "aliens," creatures from outer space, even beyond our own universe. "They" are usually assigned villain roles, intent on causing chaos to earth people. This is clearly a projection of our own destructive nature, for we have no valid reason to presume "aliens" are ill intentioned. Nevertheless, dealing with pollution, providing enough food, arming ourselves to "fight" viral and bacterial infections, cancer, prolonging our healthy life span, the threat of natural calamity such as a meteor in our path, weather extremes such as global warming, and radioactivity in our galaxy are motives for all humanity to become allied to beneficially focus our energy on establishing ANWOT.

I view the urgency for the development of ANWOT more than an opportunity; it is a requirement for our survival. Though we grow in sophistication, our core remains dedicated to *fight or flight*. And our middle "nurtured" layer has devised a mental O.S. that converts physical attack to symbolic means of control; when agreements, treaties, and the symbols of preferred consequences fail, we regularly fall back to physical means of domination, including war. As we attempt to create the means of function that supports globalization and communal well-being, we best not forget that we have not shed our more primitive behaviors. They are prominently exhibited in our history <u>and</u> our present, and we can expect they will be ever with us. Our personal task is to educate our "outer" mental layer of *self*-mastery to provide wise direction to the physical powers we have inherited and now dramatically expand.

---

[32] At the time of the 1986 Cold War, there were an estimated 70,000 nuclear warheads, and 128,000 nuclear warheads built since 1945. *Bulletin of the Atomic Scientists*, July/August, 2006, p.64.

We have advanced physical science and mastered immense power due to our labeling and classification of the electrical, chemical, biologic, and mechanical means of operation we universally share, i.e. the more visible *physical* "signals" for action. For example, scientific method has empowered us with the means to create effective physical interventions in medicine and surgery. We may readily understand the gap between our *physical* and *mental* science. The former have commonly shared fixed properties. Our brain is endowed with prewired sophisticated senses that convey the data of our physical world to our conscious awareness. By programming symbols with "meaning" to create virtual reality, we have added a new personal "second signal system" which is private and deviant of the rules universally applied to physical phenomena. We lack equivalent "senses" that identify our *mental* O.S.s, one from another, and which pathway a thought is to be processed. However, this task is as attainable as it is urgent. To direct our *mental* function as we do our *physical* function, we must devise a more practical scientific labeling system. The labeling system here provided recognizes key word-switches as members of one of three families. This minimal classification is the prerequisite to develop a science of thought management as we have developed our physical sciences.

Humankind has attained its degree of *self*-mastery by teaching our most recent-to-evolve mental capacity (1) to process information (think) using symbols to create a private personal virtual reality, (2) to *reflect* on our thoughts and thinking independent of input from our genes and nurturers, (3) to convert data into energy-laden words and concepts, and (4) to use will power, i.e. the trigger-power of symbols, to direct energy to an outcome of its (our *self's*) own design. Our *self* (*our freedom organ*) "speaks" through its mental second signaling system. It excels using mental concepts, logic, assumptions, and beliefs to influence action. Our *self's* rational problem-solving skills may direct thinking that is otherwise primarily responsive to fate and circumstance. We may view our *self* as a sort of biologic computer, unique in that **we (our reflective-thinking mental *self*) can develop the mental capacity to modify thoughts and/or initiate our own original programs! We have the ability to create a newer way of thinking, a science of thought control. We are increasingly empowering ourselves to not only master our own fate but to alter the fate of our world.**

The primary purpose I have written <u>A Newer Way of Thinking</u> is to encourage you to join me in making ANWOT education available to our populace. If we choose to divert our present course leading to the creation of our own *big bang,* we must replace *cure,* as emphasized by our prevalent manner of thinking, with *prevention.* We must attain *mental freedom* from the prejudices of nature and our nurturers through what has also been called *becoming our own person, thought control,* and/or *self-mastery.* As role models, we become an important force for peace in the world, *one* of the *"each one, teach one"* who will help popularize the needed updates to our manner of thinking.

The same technology that thrust us into this new nuclear era is ours to free our will and rapidly educate the manner we think to consistently work <u>for</u> us. <u>A Newer Way of Thinking</u> explains why and how the task is quite doable. Mass communication is now available at little or no cost, at one's own convenient place and time. You will learn why we must energize the huge majority whose passivity allows a few bigots to determine the fate of the world, and all therein we love. The mental skills that make a difference are presented in plain language, understandable by anyone capable of reading this book. I need your participation and you need ANWOT! So let's get on with making this world a kinder, gentler place for ourselves, those we love, and those we will never meet. Those readers who already possess the mental insights that lead to *feeling good* and *doing good* are invited to expand what this guide has to offer by contributing to our blog (linked to the Internet site **www.anwot.org**).

I want you to know that I have no profit motive in writing this book. You may obtain the ANWOT skills <u>FREE</u> on the Educational Community Internet site **anwot.org**. FREE means you will not be asked for money or to buy anything. You may read it on the monitor or print hard copies. I have attained financial independence so that I don't need and don't want financial gain from my endeavor. <u>A Newer Way of Thinking</u> is the product of my privileged education. The books are my attempt to fulfill my obligation to pass on the wisdom others have generously and enthusiastically shared, to give back what others have provided to me. A printed copy cannot be produced without a publisher's cost. However, I pledge that any profits will be used to further the spread of ANWOT through The Educational Community, Inc., a 501(c)(3) nonprofit corporation I have created and funded, or through another nonprofit sponsor dedicated to promoting global well-being. The printed short course is available for purchase if you prefer the convenience of reading from print rather than a monitor, because it may be more expensive to make your own hard copy, and/or you would like any profit from the published copy to benefit our mission – peace of mind and world peace. I take credit for the <u>Guide</u>'s wisdoms merely as a lifelong *collector*. My greatest satisfaction is that you the reader are willing to invest your time and energy to critically consider the validity of <u>A Newer Way of Thinking</u>. *Each one, teach one* is a powerful resource. Become *one* and make a difference! How about it? Will you join the architects and engineers that can make ANWOT happen? Enjoy becoming a valuable member of the larger community we all share as you help grow our collective wealth.

Please accept the ANWOT guide to feeling good and doing good as my gift for our personal well-being. <u>A Newer Way of Thinking</u> is a gift you can refuse, but you may regret missing this educational opportunity. To it, I urge you to add your own life's wisdom. Make it your personal gift to others!

Highlights of ANWOT Behavior "vs." Highlights of Nature/Nurture Behavior

The chart that follows contrasts the perspectives and action outcomes of behavior when information is processed substituting the ANWOT *self*-mastery manner of directing information for the passively inherited manner of thinking acquired from our genes and modified by our nurturers through our immature dependent years of development. The positives and negatives are emphasized to highlight the contrast.

HIGHLIGHTS OF ANWOT BEHAVIOR	*HIGHLIGHTS OF NATURE/NURTURE BEHAVIOR*
LOVE: I create and maintain my love-making factory. I generate love to fill my own needs and have excess to share with others. I welcome love from others.	LOVE: I am a love junkie depending on others to fulfill my requirement for love and approval. I am upset when the person(s) I need love from loves another.
AGGRESSION: I aggressively direct my energy to constructive purposes for myself and the greater community. I energetically pursue conflict resolution, win-win relationships.	AGGRESSION: I use physical and mental aggression to get my way. I must win and see to it that the "other" loses even if it is harmful to me.
POWER: Power is a useful asset when applied with wisdom. It is a tool to do constructive things.	POWER: Power helps me get my way. I want as much as I can get. I want to dominate others.
WISDOM: A fulfilled life requires wise *self*-direction. The pursuit of wisdom is a lifetime goal; I can learn much from others.	WISDOM: Power is wisdom. I know what is good and right. Those with powerful tools make the rules.
WORLD VIEW: The world is my garden. I have a choice of many things I can grow here and enjoy the outcome of my labor.	WORLD VIEW: I have been provided for in my early years. I should be taken care of during my lifetime. If I don't get what I need, it's somebody's fault.
LANGUAGE: When I can, I use descriptive words that dispose to problem-solving and analog words that provide me a more accurate picture of things.	LANGUAGE: I am used to prescriptive words that point out who's to blame and dichotomous words that make it clear which side is the good and right one.
RELATIONSHIPS: I am my lifetime traveling companion and work to become my best friend. I share my good feelings with others.	RELATIONSHIPS: Friends are important because I can get what I need from them. I am worthwhile if and when others give me praise and show me love.
PROBLEM-SOLVING: I regularly ask "What is most likely to get me what I want in the short term <u>and</u> the long term." This usually occurs with cooperation, consensus, compromise, patience, dialogue, and other skills of conflict resolution.	PROBLEM-SOLVING: I hope someone or God will resolve this problem. If I were boss, I'd know how to handle it. Much of my life though is "grinning and bearing it" because the "haves" have it and unfortunately I don't.

HIGHLIGHTS OF ANWOT BEHAVIOR (CONTINUED)	HIGHLIGHTS OF NATURE/NURTURE BEHAVIOR (CONTINUED)
ORIGINALITY, CREATIVITY: I come up with creative new ideas and methods that I determine will make a contribution to my well-being and/or that of my community.	ORIGINALITY, CREATIVITY: I come up with creative new ideas and methods that will please some important "other." I want the love and adoration that comes from doing what they say is worthwhile.
CHILD REARING: At first I need to set firm limits to direct them. As they mature, I will educate them to think for themselves and become what they choose to become.	CHILD REARING: I will teach my kids right from wrong, and demand that they make me proud. When they go astray, the right punishment will correct things.
DIRECTION: Now that I am empowered to think for myself, I am responsible for the direction of my life's experience. There are many fulfilling paths to choose from.	DIRECTION: I am stuck in what fate has made me. Others have given me a good idea what I am and what I'm suited for so I might try to make the best of it.
INDEPENDENCE, HABIT: I am my own person. I am grateful for what has been provided and now I'm master of my own ship. Consider, but don't depend on habit.	INDEPENDENCE, HABIT: What has got me this far has "worked" to a degree. The old path is what I was taught and what I know; hopefully it will work out the best.
VALUES, RELIGION: My beliefs and the meanings I ascribe to the world have largely been acquired from my nurturers. I will critically evaluate them and determine what makes sense to me.	VALUES, RELIGION: I have been educated in the ways of the world, have been told the right way to believe and how to properly act. If the authorities said it, it must be O.K. and the right thing for me.
FREEDOM: I have been provided the unique opportunity to free myself from the control of other "masters" and own my thinking and therefore my feelings and actions. I will gratefully strive to wisely direct my life's experience.	FREEDOM: As long as I do the right thing and follow the rules, I will be granted a good life's experience. By being creative and pleasing the authorities that prescribe the correct way of thinking and doing, I will be rewarded and not punished.
TOLERANCE: While I don't respect all views, I try to respect all people and promote friendship. There is plenty of room for differences of opinion.	TOLERANCE: I know who the good people are and who is trustworthy. Others need to be taught to think and act in the right way or be punished.

Although Einstein is known as "father of the bomb," he was an avid humanitarian and peacenik. He was persuaded to write the famous letter to the President of the United States that led to the Manhattan Project and the atomic bomb only after he considered what we all know would happen if Nazi Germany got there first. He spent the last ten years of his life spreading the seeds for a new way of thinking. For these seeds (and humanity) to grow into maturity, they require nourishment from a variety of individuals. I have no doubt that the collective efforts of a few committed individuals can create a huge change.

It worked for Alcoholics Anonymous, Amway cleaning products, Mary Kay cosmetics, and every major religion. A similar few can surely spread the newer way of thinking urged by the person most regard as the world's brightest mind.

This bonus section is my appeal to those who have the power to provide the needed nourishment. We have a beginning blueprint for ANWOT. We require the few **one's** of the *each one, teach one* to get the ball rolling. The most immediate need is from persons who influence the media: promoters of radio and T.V., editors of newspapers and magazines, persons knowledgeable about the Internet who can harness this powerful new means for the greater good, and sales persons of all kind. You of the media control the resources that can inspire others who will further lead the way. Talented writers, cartoonists, graphic designers, and the multitude of creative individuals whose imagination can make a difference are needed to convey the basic message in the language that is understood by the diverse segments of our population: perhaps a comic book for children, an "orientation" course for college students, a translation for specific language groups, an educational format for the human services worker within the corporate world. If the initial steps are successful, I foresee our community's "haves" will become motivated to more freely invest their wealth to educate the "have nots."

If not now, when? Do you hear the ALARM clock? It is time to wake up. Our scientists have told us the Doomsday Clock is ticking. We have the collective wisdom to reverse the clock. Yes, a few can start the process, but you are needed to sustain the momentum. Most know the adage: "Give a hungry person a fish and he will eat for a day; teach him to fish and he will eat the rest of his life." It is time we focus our resources on educating our population in ANWOT so that those we love will live their life and enjoy the wishes we make for them. Take the first steps. Become your own best friend and your own genie through a newer way of thinking. Enriching yourself with mental wealth will help make our most universal wishes a reality.

This bonus section of <u>The Short Course to Mental Wealth</u> explains why the talents of many persons with diverse skills are needed if we are to survive and thrive in the new Nuclear Age. You have received food for thought. Thought stimulates thinking. Thinking may serve as a preparation for action or a substitution for action. Which will you choose?

RAISE FUNDS FOR YOUR NONPROFIT CORPORATION

NON-PROFIT ORGANIZATIONS: If you are a charitable group dedicated to making the world a safer more wonder place, The Educational Community, Inc. (**E.C.**) will sell **The Short Course to Mental Wealth** or **A Newer Way of Thinking** (when published) to you in quantity at our cost. Keep ALL of the profits. That's not a mistake – 100% of the profits!

FOR-PROFIT GROUPS: Every organization with a social conscience, whatever their identified mission, welcomes the opportunity to participate in solving our greatest immediate threat to well-being – destructive aggression. **Mental Wealth's** curriculum of practical wisdoms is applicable to all religions, *peaceniks*, corporate human service programs, and professional offices. **Mental Wealth** builds company moral and is a marvelous image builder creating customer appreciation. It enriches individuals AND our global community. Buy in quantity and the E. C. will donate 100% of its profits to the charitable organization of the sponsor's choice.

HOW COME? NOBODY GIVES AWAY 100% OF THEIR PROFITS.

Drastic issues require drastic measures. We require fast action. Einstein, the person commonly identified as the world's brightest mind AND our most respected and knowledgeable scientists have diagnosed a new community cancer that is rapidly spreading, will attack our loved ones with little or no warning, is so virulent that it rapidly kills, and our only defense is prevention. Extreme incentives to rapidly educate ourselves in a newer manner of thinking are justified when the stakes are ultimate. Every weapon that has ever been developed has been used to its fullest. How many H-bombs can we afford?

We began the road to civilization 50,000 years ago. The wonderful news is that we now have the knowledge AND the powerful mass media to complete the task. Popularizing the newer way of thinking is our best hope to significantly and rapidly change ourselves; each person who acquires the love and wisdom that is ours for the making takes our world to a kinder gentler place.

The Educational Community, Inc. receives its support from retail sales of its products and unsolicited voluntary contributions. Action is required more than money.

For more information: email: ddpet@comcast.net   Mark E-mail "**E.C. query**"

The Educational Community, Inc.
c/o Donald Pet, M.D.
235 East River Drive, Unit 1107
East Hartford, CT 06108

Never doubt that a small group of thoughtful, committed citizens can change the world. Indeed, it is the only thing that ever has.   **Margaret Mead**